AYURVEDA AND THE MIND

the Healing *of* Consciousness

DAVID FRAWLEY

LOTUS
PRESS

DISCLAIMER

This book is not intended to treat, diagnose or prescribe. The information contained herein is in no way to be considered as a substitute for a consultation with a duly licensed health care professional.

Editor: Parvati Markus
Cover art and design: Paul Bond, Art & Soul Design
Illustrations: Margo Gal & Angela Werneke
Design & Page Layout: Carola Höchst-Teague

First Edition   1997
Fourth Printing   2011
Fifth Printing   2015
Sixth Printing   2019

Printed in the United States of America

Library of Congress Cataloging-in-Publication-Data
Ayurveda and the Mind, The Healing of Consciousness
includes bibliographical references.
ISBN: 978-0-9149-5536-8   96-80088
                                                CIP

Published by:
Lotus Press, P.O. Box 325, Twin Lakes, WI 53181 USA
web: www.lotuspress.com
Email: lotuspress@lotuspress.com
800.824.6396

ACKNOWLEDGEMENTS

I wish to thank various teachers and their work who have provided inspiration for the book. These include Swami Yogeshwaranda, Ganapati Muni, Rishi Daivarata, Sri Aurobindo, Sri Anirvan, and Ram Swarup and the perennial yogic and Vedic tradition which they represent. I must also honor all great yogis and Ayurvedic doctors who have developed, preserved and passed on this science throughout the millennia.

I want to especially thank Lenny Blank for organizing the production of the book in such an expeditious manner, and Dr. David Simon, not only for his Foreword but for his ongoing encouragement and special interest in this aspect of my work.

TABLE OF CONTENTS

Foreword

Preface

Part I 1
Ayurvedic Psychology: Yogic Mind-Body Medicine

1. A New Journey into Consciousness.........................3

2. Ayurvedic Constitutional Types: The Biological
   Humors of Vata, Pitta and Kapha.........................11

3. The Three Gunas: How to Balance Your
   Consciousness 29

4. The Nature of the Mind 43

5. The Five Elements and the Mind 59

Part II 73
The Energetics of Consciousness

6. Conditioned Consciousness:
   The Greater Mental Field 75

7. Intelligence: The Power of Perception 93

8. The Outer Mind: The Field of the Senses 109

9. Ego and Self: The Quest for Identity 125

Part III 147
Ayurvedic Therapies for the Mind

10. Ayurvedic Counseling and
    Behavioral Modification 149

11. The Cycle of Nutrition for the Mind:
The Role of Impressions 169

12. Outer Treatment Modalities:
Diet, Herbs, Massage and Pancha Karma 187

13. Subtle Therapies:
Colors, Gems and Aromas...................................205

14. The Healing Power of Mantra 223

Part IV 241

Spiritual Applications: Yoga and Ayurvedic Psychology

15. Spiritual Therapies 243

16. The Eightfold Method of Yoga I:
Outer Practices 259

17. The Eightfold Method of Yoga II:
Inner Practices 279

Appendix 1: Tables...307

A. The Three Bodies 307

B. Five Sheaths and the Mind 309

C. Seven Levels of the Universe 311

D. The Seven Chakras 312

E. The Five Pranas and the Mind 314

F. Table of Functions of the Mind.........................317

Appendix 2..319

Footnotes 319

Sanskrit Glossary 326

Herbal Glossary 329

Bibliography..332

About the Author 334

Index 336

FOREWORD

Human beings face unprecedented challenges as we approach the next millennium. We are seeking new ways to meet the demands of modern life as its unrelenting flow of information demands our attention. Although in many ways, we have greater opportunities for a rich and fulfilling life than ever before, it is clear that we need to evolve new strategies if we are to survive and thrive as individuals and as a species.

Our Western culture is dynamic, vibrant, and eagerly embraces change. Our enthusiasm for that which is new enables us to cross technological and philosophical boundaries that were unimaginable a century ago. Yet, this fascination with change has extracted a toll on our society. Many people feel uprooted, disconnected from the great traditions that have provided guidance and nourishment to human beings for thousands of years.

The ancient Vedic tradition, cognized by the great seers of India, willingly offers us a wealth of practical knowledge on how to live a healthy and meaningful life. Vedic wisdom is timeless and unbounded and, therefore, it is relevant in this modern age. Fortunately, we have Dr. David Frawley to translate and interpret this profound information so it can be transformed into living knowledge for all who ingest it.

In his latest book, *Ayurveda and the Mind,* Dr. Frawley once again shines his brilliant intellectual light to illuminate the practical applications of Ayurveda and Yoga as applied to the mind. Through his clear exposition of the Vedic principles of consciousness and its expressions, a simple, yet profound approach to psychological and emotional healing is elucidated. This book reminds us that the mind is a subtle organ, whose health depends upon its ability to extract nourishment from the environment. If we have accumulated toxicity in the form of emotional wounds, frustrations, disappointments or wrong beliefs, eliminating these impurities from our mental and emotional layers is essential if we are to have true emotional and spiritual freedom.

Unlike modern psychological science which has until very recently maintained the dichotomy of mind and body, Ayurvedic psychology clearly recognizes that the mind and the body are one. The mind is a field of ideas, the body is a field of molecules, but both are expressions of consciousness interacting with itself.

This book is a valuable resource to students of Ayurveda, Yoga, Tantra and psychology. Dr. Frawley has again demonstrated his unique talent of digesting ancient Vedic knowledge and feeding us this understanding, which nourishes our body, mind and soul. He has been a dear and true teacher to me and I feel great appreciation for the loving wisdom he so readily shares with me and the world.

David Simon, M.D.
Medical Director, The Chopra Center for Well-Being
La Jolla, California

PREFACE

Ayurveda is the extraordinary mind-body medicine of India with its great yogic spiritual
tradition, a tremendous resource for bringing
wholeness to all levels of our existence. It is one of the
world's oldest and most complete systems of natural healing, containing great wisdom for all humanity that all of
us should know.

The present volume examines the psychological aspect
of Ayurveda, which is probably the most important part of
the system and the least understood. This book goes into
the Ayurvedic view of the mind and its relationship with
both body and spirit, which is profound and intricate. It
outlines a comprehensive Ayurvedic treatment for the
mind, both for promoting health and for dealing with disease, using diverse methods from diet to meditation.

These teachings derive from classical Ayurvedic texts,
which commonly contain sections on the mind and its
treatment. They also relate to yogic teachings, from which
Ayurveda derives its view of consciousness and many of its
modalities for treating the mind. However, I have not only
examined the traditional psychological teachings of
Ayurveda, I have also tried to make them relevant to the
modern world. Ayurveda, as the science of life, is not a
frozen science but one that grows with the movement of
life itself, of which it partakes.

Plan of the Book

This book does not require that the reader possess prior knowledge of Ayurveda, though this is certainly helpful. It introduces the basic factors of Ayurveda, like the biological humors (doshas), particularly as related to psychology. On this foundation, however, the book does go deeply into its subject. It aims at providing the reader with sufficient knowledge to use the information and techniques of Ayurveda to improve his or her own life and consciousness on all levels. It is not simply introductory in nature and should be relevant to psychologists and therapists as well.

I am not going to apologize for producing a more technical book on Ayurveda than the beginning reader might understand. There are already a number of introductory books on Ayurveda that can be examined for those who require this. Now there is a need for more advanced books to unfold this important subject further. Something of the depths of Ayurveda needs to be revealed to complement the general introductions now available.

This book is divided into four sections, followed by an appendix:

Part I. Ayurvedic Psychology: Yogic Mind-Body Medicine

Part II. The Energetics of Consciousness

Part III. Ayurvedic Therapies for the Mind

Part IV. Spiritual Applications of Ayurvedic Psychology: The Paths of Yoga

Appendices

The first section explains the Ayurvedic view of the mind and body and how they function. It begins with the basic material of the three gunas (Sattva, Rajas and Tamas), the three biological humors (Vata, Pitta and Kapha), and the five elements (earth, water, fire, air and ether), show-ing their relationship with the mind. It also explores the nature and functions of the mind in a general way from an Ayurvedic perspective.

The second section continues with an in-depth exami-nation of the different functions of awareness through con-sciousness, intelligence, mind, ego and self. This presents a deeper and more detailed understanding of the mind than in modern psychology, examining all layers of the mind from the subconscious to the superconscious.

In the third section of the book, we examine various Ayurvedic therapies for the mind. These begin with Ayurvedic counseling methods and the Ayurvedic view of how to treat the mind. Therapies are twofold: outer and inner. Outer therapies are linked with physical modalities like diet, herbs and massage. Inner therapies work through impressions and consist mainly of color, aroma and mantra therapies.

The fourth section of the book deals with spiritual and yogic practices from an Ayurvedic and psychological per-spective and summarizes and integrates all the therapies given in the previous section. This allows us to use the wisdom of Ayurveda not only for physical and mental health, but also for spiritual growth. The appendix con-tains various tables on the functions of the mind and their correspondences. Footnotes, glossaries, bibliography and index follow at the end.

The material in *Ayurveda and the Mind* reflects and builds on that presented in my previous books. There is a chapter on Ayurveda and the mind in my book *Ayurvedic Healing: A Comprehensive Guide.* The nature of conscious-ness, from a more spiritual and meditative perspective, is examined in *Beyond The Mind.* The present volume falls in between these two books. It has points in common with *Tantric Yoga and the Wisdom Goddesses: Spiritual Secrets of Ayurveda*, which deals with the chakras and the energetics of the subtle body. The reader can look into these books for more information on the greater system of which this book is but a part.

It is my wish that this book will stimulate more research into the psychological side of Ayurveda and its interface with the science of Yoga. This will add an important new dimension in health and human understanding for the coming century.

May the minds of all beings find peace!
May all the worlds find peace!

Dr. David Frawley
(Vamadeva Shastri)
October 1996

The Origin of Consciousness in the Heart

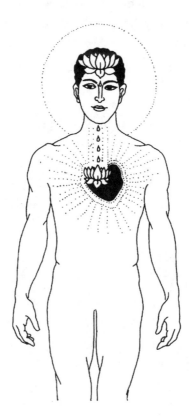

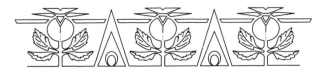

Part I

Ayurvedic Psychology: Yogic Mind-Body Medicine

In this initial section we will introduce the main concepts of Ayurvedic psychology for easy understanding of what will follow later in the book. We begin with the biological humors of Vata (air), Pitta (fire), and Kapha (water). These are the basis for determining both physical and psychological constitution. Then follows a discussion of the three qualities (gunas) of Sattva, Rajas and Tamas, which determine mental and spiritual nature. This section contains two practical self-examination tests. A test for Ayurvedic constitution concludes the chapter on constitution and one for mental nature concludes the chapter on the gunas. Readers should take these tests in order to use the material in the book in a personal way.

Then we move to the nature and functions of the mind through the five elements of earth, water, fire, air and ether. This presents an energetic approach to the mind following a similar model to Vata, Pitta and Kapha for the body. These chapters contain several practical exercises for the reader to examine how his or her own mind is working. But we begin with an introduction and overview to our vast subject.

1. A New Journey Into Consciousness

In this book we will embark upon a great inner adventure. We will journey into the different dimensions of our consciousness, individual and cosmic, known and unknown. Yet our approach will not proceed through mere imagination or speculation, nor will we leave the ground on which we stand. We will explore an integral view of the mind that includes the physical body on one side and our immortal Self on the other. We will look into all aspects of our nature and how they affect how we think, feel, perceive and are aware.

For this journey we will employ the wisdom of the great yogis and rishis of the Himalayas. This yogic wisdom is not mere technical know-how, philosophical profundity, or religious revelation. It is the wisdom of Life itself beyond any opinions or dogmas. For this you, the reader, must participate. You yourself must become both the observer and the observed. To truly probe into the mind is to journey into one's own Being. It is to explore not merely our surface time-bound ego, but our true Self, of which all that we see, internally and externally, is but a reflection. You will discover all the forces of Nature working within you, and that you yourself are a replica of the cosmos, with your inner consciousness one with God.

Ayurveda

Ayurveda is the five thousand year old Vedic "Science of Life," the traditional natural healing system of India. It is the medical side of the yogic systems of the Indian sub-continent that have included Yoga, Vedanta, Tantra and Buddhism. Today Ayurveda is at the forefront of mind-body medicine. It has spread far beyond its traditional base and is gaining attention throughout the world. Ancient Ayurveda, with its understanding of life and conscious-ness, does not appear archaic or obsolete but a key to the medicine of the future. This is because of the unique and spiritual way that Ayurveda views our place in the uni-verse.

Ayurveda views the physical body as a crystallization of deep-seated mental tendencies carried over from previous lives. It regards the mind as the reflection of the body and the storehouse of the impressions we access through the senses. It recognizes our true Self and immortal nature beyond the mind-body complex, in which we can tran-scend all physical and mental difficulties. Ayurveda com-prehends body, mind and spirit in a single view and has specific methods for working on each.

Ayurveda does not look upon the human being as a limited set of biochemical processes. It does not regard the mind as merely a function of the brain. It does not look upon the individual as a product of social circumstances, though all these factors can be important. Ayurveda views the human soul as pure awareness, linked with but not limited to the mind-body complex, which is its instru-ment of manifestation.

The body itself is a mental organism, a vehicle of per-ception designed to support the functions of the senses and to facilitate experience by the mind. Any breakdown in bodily function has its root in the perceptual process and results from wrong use of the senses. Too much, too little or wrong use of the senses results in wrong actions that cause us eventual pain. To understand how our body functions, we must also see how we use our minds.

Yoga, Ayurveda and Tantra

Ayurveda is the healing branch of yogic science. Yoga is the spiritual aspect of Ayurveda, while Ayurveda is the therapeutic branch of Yoga. Yoga is far more than the asana or exercise aspect of Yoga that is most visible in the West today. Yoga in its original intention is a science of spiritual development aiming at Self-realization, the discovery of our true nature beyond time and space. This process is aided by a mind and body free from disease.

Yoga as a medical therapy[1] is traditionally part of Ayurveda, which deals with the treatment of both physical and mental diseases. Ayurveda uses yogic methods, like Yoga postures and breathing exercises, to treat physical diseases.[2] Ayurvedic treatment methods for the mind include yogic practices for spiritual growth, like mantra and meditation. The Ayurvedic view of the mind derives from Yoga philosophy and its understanding of the different levels of consciousness.[3] Ayurvedic and Yoga psychology were thus originally the same and have only recently begun to diverge. This is because people, particularly in the West, including Yoga teachers, do not always know the connection between Yoga and Ayurveda.

There are a number of approaches called Yoga psychology in the world today. Some of these combine Yoga postures with the methods of psychoanalysis. Some combine yogic meditation methods with Western psychiatric or medical approaches. Others use yogic methods directly to heal the mind but without reference to Ayurveda. These approaches can be useful but work better when combined with Ayurveda, which is the original yogic healing approach and provides the proper medical language for using Yoga fully as a healing science.

Ayurveda and Yoga both relate to the system of Tantra, which provides various techniques for changing the nature of consciousness. However, true Tantra is much more than its current popular idea as a system of sexual practices that reflects only a small and generally lower aspect of Tantra. Tantra is a complete system of human development that can aid us in improving all aspects of our lives.

Tantric tools include sensory therapies of color, gems, sounds and mantras, along with the use of various deities. Deities, like Shiva or the Divine Mother, are archetypes which can bring about changes at a depth in consciousness that the personal mind cannot reach. Sensory therapies change what we put into the mind, which can alter negative conditioning without the need for analysis. Ayurvedic methods for healing the mind include Tantra. The Tantric understanding of the subtle forces of mind and body also relates to Ayurveda. Most deeper yogic approaches also employ such higher Tantric methods.

Mind-Body Medicine

Ayurvedic doctors need not call themselves psychologists. Psychology is part of their usual practice that considers both physical and mental disease. According to Ayurveda, physical diseases occur mainly owing to external factors like wrong diet or exposure to pathogens. Mental diseases arise mainly from internal factors, like wrong use of the senses and the accumulation of negative emotions. These follow our karma, the results of our past actions that comes from previous lives. However, both physical and psychological diseases are usually mixed and one seldom occurs without the other.

Some diseases, like acute infections, have almost entirely physical causes and can be treated purely on a physical level. However, most diseases have psychological causes and all lasting diseases have psychological effects. Physical disease disturbs the emotions and weakens the senses, which may give rise to psychological disturbances. Psychological imbalances have physical consequences. They lead to dietary indiscretions, strain the heart and nerves, and weaken the physical body.

In the modern developed world, our problems are mainly psychological. We have adequate food, clothing and shelter, which prevents us from getting most physical diseases. Yet, though most of us have no major physical problems, we still suffer from psychological unrest. This unrest may manifest as feelings of loneliness, not being loved or appreciated, anger, stress, or anxiety. It can lead to the weakening of our physical energy and prevent us from doing what we really want to do.

Our very way of life breeds unhappiness. We have an active and turbulent culture in which there is little peace or contentment. We have disturbed the organic roots of life, which are good food, water and air, and a happy family life. We live in an artificial world dominated by an urban landscape and mass media, in which there is little to nourish the soul. We ever desire new things and are seldom content with what we have. We run from one stimulation to another, rarely observing the process of our lives that is really leading nowhere. Our lives are patterns of accumulation in which we are never still or at rest. Our medicine is more a quick fix to keep us going in our wrong lifestyles and seldom addresses the behavioral root of our problems. We take a quick pill hoping that our problem will go away, not recognizing that it may only be a symptom of a life out of balance, like a warning light that we had better heed.

Ayurveda, on the other hand, teaches harmony with Nature, simplicity and contentment as keys to well-being. It shows us how to live in a state of balance in which fulfillment is a matter of being, not becoming. It connects us with the wellsprings of creativity and happiness within our own consciousness, so that we can permanently overcome our psychological problems. Ayurveda provides a real solution to our health problems, which is to return to oneness with both the universe and the Divine within. This requires changing how we live, think and perceive.

Levels of Ayurvedic Healing

Ayurveda recognizes four primary levels of healing:
1. Disease Treatment
2. Disease Prevention
3. Life Enhancement
4. Awareness Development

For most of us, medical treatment begins when we fall ill. It is a form of disease treatment, a response to a condition that has already occurred. It aims at fixing something already broken. However, if medicine begins with the treatment of disease, it is a failure because the disease is already harming us. At this late stage, radical and invasive methods may be required, like drugs or surgery, which have many side effects.

A higher level of healing is to eliminate diseases before they manifest, for which invasive methods like drugs or surgery are seldom necessary. To reach this stage we must consider the effects our lifestyle, environment, work and psychological condition. We must cut off the wrong factors in our daily lives that make us vulnerable to disease.

To some extent we are always sick because life itself is transient and unstable. There is always some disease attacking us, particularly in changes of season or in the aging process. Each creature that is born must eventually die. Health is a matter of continual adjustment, like sailing a ship upon the sea. It cannot be permanently achieved and then forgotten, but is an ongoing concern.

The third level of treatment is life-enhancement therapy, which aims at improving our vitality and enabling us to live longer. It does not merely prevent diseases but shows us how to increase our positive vitality. However, Ayurveda aims at more than merely creating health, avoiding disease and helping us live longer.

The fourth level of Ayurveda is awareness development. This requires a spiritual approach to life, including meditation. To be healthy is important but health is not an end in itself. It is not enough merely to prolong our lives and have better energy to do the things we want. We must consider what we are using our energy for and why. The quality of our awareness is the real fruit of all that we do. It is our ultimate expression, the essence of who we really are. Our awareness is the only thing that we can take with us when we die. It can continue growing as the body and mind decline and is our greatest aid in the aging process.

The purpose of physical incarnation is to help develop a higher consciousness. This not only lifts us individually but raises the world and the rest of humanity. All our human problems arise from lack of true awareness, which is not merely a lack of information but a failure to understand our place in the universe. Actually we do not have a place in the universe at all. The universe rests within us. The entire universe is part of our own greater being.

All human beings are part of our own Self. All creatures are but different forms of who we are. They are like the different leaves and branches of the tree of consciousness. True awareness is the recognition of unity through which we transcend personal limitations and understand the Self as All. This is the ultimate goal of Ayurveda, which aims at releasing us from all sorrow and suffering. True awareness is the ultimate cure for all psychological disorders. But to understand it we must first look into the mind and its functions. We must start where we are. In this direction, our journey proceeds.

2. Ayurvedic Constitutional Types: The Biological Humors of Vata, Pitta and Kapha

If we look at the different people in the world around us, we observe that all of us are not simply alike. The standard or average person is a statistical abstraction who does not really exist. Each one of us is different in many ways, both physically and mentally. Each person possesses a unique constitution different from that of any other person. The shapes and sizes, temperaments and characters of people have enormous variations that must affect our health and happiness.

We must understand our own nature for our own happiness and well-being in life. Similarly, we must understand the nature of others, which may be different than our own, for harmonious social interaction. The food that is good for one person may not be good for another. One person may thrive on spices, for example, while another similar person may not be able to tolerate them. Similarly, the psychological conditions favorable for one person may not suit another. Competition may stimulate one person to greater achievement but intimidate another and make him fail.

Without understanding our particular constitution, we must fall into poor health and disease. No standardized medicine can adequately deal with all our individual variations. Only a system that can discern our different constitutional types has this capacity. Ayurveda contains such a well-developed science of individual types as its core wisdom. One of the great beauties of Ayurveda is that it so clearly helps us understand all our individual variations, special abilities and idiosyncrasies.

However, human constitutional patterns fall into general categories and do not occur at random. While these have variations, they occur in well-defined groups, mirroring the great forces of Nature. Three major constitutional types exist according to the three biological humors that are the root forces of our physical life. These are called Vata, Pitta and Kapha in Sanskrit, which correspond to the three great elements of air, fire and water as they function in the mind-body complex. Ayurvedic books emphasize the physical aspects of these three types. Here we will give more attention to their psychological ramifications. Let us first introduce Vata, Pitta and Kapha and how they function.

Vata — Air

The biological air-humor is called Vata, which means literally "what blows," referring to the wind. It contains a secondary aspect of ether as the field in which it moves. The spaces in the head, joints and bones serve as its containers.

Vata governs movement and is responsible for the discharge of all impulses both voluntary and involuntary. It works mainly through the brain and nervous system. In the digestive system, it relates to the lower abdomen, particularly the large intestine where gas (air) accumulates. The senses of touch and hearing, which correspond to the air and ether elements, are part of it. Vata is the force that directs and guides the other humors because life itself derives from air. Vata allows for agility, adaptability and facility in action. Its power animates us and makes us feel vital and enthusiastic.

Vata rules the basic sensitivity and mobility of the mental field. It energizes all mental functions from the senses to the subconscious. It allows us to respond mentally to external and internal impulses. Fear and anxiety are its prime emotional derangements, which occur when we feel our life-force is somehow threatened or jeopardized.

Pitta — Fire

The biological fire-humor is called Pitta, which means "what cooks." Fire cannot exist directly in the body but is held in hot liquids like the blood and digestive fluids. For this reason, Pitta contains a secondary aspect of water.

Pitta governs transformation in the body and mind as digestion and assimilation on all levels from food to ideas. It predominates in the digestive system, particularly in the small intestine and liver, where the digestive fire operates. It is also found in the blood and in the sense of sight that corresponds to the fire element. Pitta is responsible for all heat and light from sensory perception down to cellular metabolism.

Mentally, Pitta governs reason, intelligence, and understanding — the illuminating capacity of the mind. It allows the mind to perceive, judge and discriminate. Anger is its main emotional disturbance, which is fiery, heats us up, and helps us defend ourselves from external attacks.

Kapha — Water

The biological water-humor is called Kapha, literally "what sticks." It contains a secondary aspect of earth as the boundary in which it is held, the skin and mucous membranes.

Kapha governs form and substance and is responsible for weight, cohesion and stability. It is the fluid solution, the internal ocean, in which the other two humors move, and constitutes the main substance of the body. It provides for proper lubrication and discharge of secretions and cushions the nerves, mind and senses. Kapha predominates in the bodily tissues and in the upper part of the body — the stomach, lungs and head where mucus accumulates. It relates to the senses of taste and smell, which correspond to water and earth.

Kapha governs feeling, emotion, and the capacity of the mind to hold on to form. It gives mental calm and stability but can prevent growth and expansion. Desire and attachment are its main emotional imbalances, the holding on to things in the mind, which can overburden the psyche.

Feeling Vata, Pitta and Kapha

The following exercise shows how Vata, Pitta and Kapha function through the conditions of nature. Note these characteristics and try to see them in the changing conditions and climates around you.

VATA: Sit outdoors in a quiet place on a cool, dry, clear windy day, such as is common in the autumn when the leaves are falling and the first frost has occurred. Preferably find a hilly or mountain area where you have some view. Note your reaction to the environment and its qualities. At first you will feel light, clear, dry and expansive. If you remain out in the open, exposed to the wind for some time, you will eventually feel unsettled, ungrounded, vulnerable and exposed.

PITTA: Sit out in the open on a hot, muggy, partly overcast summer day. Again note your reaction to the environment. You will feel warm, moist and enveloped, perhaps pleasant in the beginning. In not too long a time, you will begin to feel hot or stuffy and will want to move indoors or do something to cool down. You may gradually become irritable or angry.

 KAPHA: Sit outdoors, in a protected place if necessary, on a cool rainy day, when the wind is calm, preferably in the spring when new vegetation is bursting forth. Note your reaction to the environment. You will first feel cool and moist, calm and content, and perhaps want to rest or sleep. After a while you will begin to feel stagnant, heavy, and resistant, unable to move. Your senses themselves may become cloudy or heavy.

Constitutional Types

The following are typical physical and psychological profiles for the three types. They need not be taken rigidly; it is the predominance of characteristics that matters.

VATA (AIR TYPES)

Physical Characteristics

Those in whom Vata, the biological air-humor, predominates are taller or shorter than average, thin in build, and have difficulty holding weight. Their frame is bony, without well-developed muscles and with prominent veins. Their skin is dry and easily becomes rough, cracked or wrinkled. Their complexion is dull or dusky with possible brown or black discoloration. Their eyes are usually small, dry and may twitch or tremor. Their hair and scalp are dry and they easily get dandruff or split ends.

Air types possess variable and fluctuating digestive powers. Their appetite may be high at times, while low or absent at others. Emotional upset, stress, or hostility quickly gives them nervous indigestion. They are light sleepers and suffer from insomnia, which may become chronic. Once disturbed, they do not fall back to sleep easily. They have restless dreams and possibly nightmares.

Relative to their waste materials, their urine is scanty and they seldom perspire much. Their stool tends to be dry and not large in quantity. They frequently get constipation, abdominal distention and gas. They most commonly suffer from pain disorders, from common headaches to chronic diseases like arthritis. Cold, wind and dryness are the main environmental factors that disturb them. Yet any extremes bother them, including too much heat or sunlight. They do not like anything harsh. Generally they do best with a warm and damp environment and a rich and nutritive diet. A nurturing and supportive emotional atmosphere is required to make them feel at peace.

Vata types are physically active and energetic. They enjoy speed, motion and aerobic activity. Yet they tire easily and lack long-term stamina and endurance. They are often athletic in youth, but lack the physique for strong exercise or contact sports. They easily get muscle spasms or stiffness. They are not entirely present in their bodies and may be clumsy. Their bones are more likely to break than other types and they are prone to injury.

Psychological Characteristics

Vata types are quick and agile in their minds with

changing interests and inclinations. They are talkative, informed, and intellectual and can understand many different points of view. However, they can be superficial in their ideas and talk on aimlessly. Their minds easily waver and can wander out of control. While they may have some knowledge of many different things, they can lack deep knowledge of a particular subject. Their will is usually indecisive and unsteady. They lack determination, consistency and self-confidence and often have negative images of themselves.

Vatas suffer most from fear, which is their first reaction to anything new or strange. They like to worry, easily get afflicted by anxiety, and usually lack stability. They get spaced out and may be absent-minded. Their memory is short-term or erratic. They suffer quickly from overwork and over-exercise and tend to overextend themselves in whatever they do.

Air types make good teachers, computer programmers and excel at communication, as with the mass media. They are good at thinking, writing and organizing data. They make good musicians but may be over-sensitive to noise. Generally, they are creative and most artists are of this type.

They can be highly sociable and like to mix with people of all types. Yet when the air element is too high, they become loners, hypersensitive to human contact. This is because they have too much to say and do not know how to relate it, not because they are really of a solitary nature. They are commonly rebels and do not like to be either leaders or followers. However, they are also the most flexible, adaptable and able to change of the three types once they understand what they need to do.

PITTA (FIRE TYPES)

Physical Characteristics

Pitta types are usually of average height and build, with well-developed muscles. Their skin is oily and has good color, but is prone to acne, rashes and other inflammatory conditions. Similarly, their eyes easily get red or inflamed. They are sensitive to sunlight and often have to wear glasses. Their hair is thin, and they commonly get early gray or balding.

Fire types usually possess an appetite that is good, sharp or excessive. They can eat most anything and not gain weight (until they get over forty). However, they are prone to hyperacidity and heartburn and may develop ulcers or hypertension. Their sleep is moderate in duration but can get disturbed, particularly by emotional conflict. They have an average amount of dreams, which may be colorful and dramatic, possibly violent.

Their bodily discharges — feces, urine or mucus — are generally yellow in color and large in quantity because their excess bile (Pitta) colors these. They are prone to loose stool or diarrhea. They sweat easily and their sweat and other discharges may be malodorous. Their blood is hot and they bruise and bleed easily. Fire-types most commonly suffer from fevers, infections, toxic blood conditions, and inflammations. They are intolerant of heat, sunlight, fire and chemicals and prefer coolness, water and shade.

Pittas are competitive and easily take to exercise or sports. They love to win and hate to lose, and enjoy games of all types. Their endurance is moderate but they tire easily under sunlight and heat. Their joints tend to be loose. Their energy and endurance are moderate but they can easily push themselves by their strong determination that may lead to exhaustion.

Psychological Characteristics

Pitta types are intelligent, perceptive and discriminating. They have sharp minds and see the world in a clear and systematic manner. Yet, because their ideas are sharp, they may be opinionated, judgmental or self-righteous. They are prone to anger, which is their main reaction to new or unexpected events, and tend to be aggressive or domineering. They have strong wills and can be impulsive or self-willed. They make good leaders but can be fanatic or insensitive. They like the use of energy and force and are prone toward argument or violence.

Pittas make good scientists and often have a good understanding of mechanics and mathematics. They like to work with tools, weapons, or chemistry. They have probing minds and are good at research and invention. They may be good psychologists and have deep insight. Most military persons or police officers are fire-types. They like law and order and see the value of punishment. Most lawyers, with their sharp minds and debating skills, are of this type, including most politicians.

Pittas are good orators or preachers and are convincing in presenting their cases. However, they may lack compassion and have a hard time seeing other points of view. They prefer hierarchy and authority over consensus and democracy. The hard-driving executive who gets a sudden heart attack is usually a high Pitta type. The same determination can serve them well, if directed to the proper goal.

KAPHA (WATER TYPES)

Physical Characteristics

Kapha types are usually shorter than normal in height and stocky in build, with well-developed chests. Occasionally they are tall but they always possess a large frame. They tend toward corpulence or obesity and hold excess weight and water unless they work hard to prevent it. Their skin is thick and tends to be damp and oily. Their eyes are large, white and attractive, with big lashes. Their hair is abundant, oily and thick. Their teeth are large, white and attractive.

Kaphas have a low but constant appetite, with a slow metabolism. They are constant but not heavy eaters and enjoy having food around them more than eating a lot. Often it is hard for them to lose weight, even if they do not eat much. They like sweets and may develop diabetes later in life. They sleep easily, often excessively, and have a hard time staying awake late into the night.

Their discharges of urine, sweat and feces are average. They can sweat a lot if they become hot, but it will come on slowly. They accumulate and discharge large amounts of mucus, particularly in the morning. Kaphas as water suffer most from diseases of excess weight or water. These include obesity, congestive disorders, swollen glands, asthma, edema and tumors (generally benign). They suffer from cold, dampness and stagnant air. They prefer heat, light, dryness and wind.

Kaphas like to be sedentary but possess strong endurance and, once active, can continue and accomplish a lot. They win more by consistency and perseverance than by speed, skill or cunning. They suffer physically mainly from inaction and lack of discipline.

Psychological Characteristics

Kapha types are emotional in temperament and, positively, have much love, devotion and loyalty. Negatively, they have much desire, attachment and may be possessive or greedy. They are romantic, sentimental, and cry easily.

Mentally, they are slower in learning than the other types but retain what they learn. Much repetition is needed for them to grasp things. They are not creative or inventive but do carry things out and make them useful. They are better at finishing things than at starting them. They like to bring things into form and create institutions and establishments.

Water-types are traditional or conventional in their behavior and beliefs. They like to belong, to be part of a group, and seldom rebel. They are good followers and prefer to work in association. They are content and accept things as they are. They are stable but sometimes stagnate. They do not like to change and find change difficult, even when they want to. They are friendly, particularly with people they know, and hold closely to their families. Yet they have difficulties relating to strangers or foreigners. While they do not like to hurt others, they may be insensitive to the needs of those outside their sphere. Sometimes they throw their weight around and smother or suppress others.

Kaphas are usually good parents and providers. In women, they make good mothers and wives and like cooking, baking and homemaking. The men may be chefs or work in restaurants. With their large chests, good lungs and good voices, they make good singers. They like to accumulate wealth and hold firmly to what they get. They excel at real estate and make good bankers. Once motivated, they can be consistent and hard workers who hold on to all that they get.

Constitutional Examination

How To Determine Your Unique Psycho-physical Nature

Each one of us possesses all three biological humors. However, their proportion varies according to the individual. One humor will usually predominate and make its characteristic mark upon our disposition.

Some individuals are strongly of one type. These are called pure Vata (pure air), pure Pitta (pure fire) and pure Kapha (pure water) types. Mixed types occur as when two or more humors stand in equal proportion. Three different dual types exist as Vata-Pitta (air-fire), Vata-Kapha (air-water) and Pitta-Kapha (fire-water). An even type in which all three humors are in balance, or VPK type, is also found, making seven major types in all.

Note which humor you check the most; this will usually indicate your constitution (though it is helpful to consult an Ayurvedic practitioner to make sure). Also remember that even when you fall clearly into one category, you will have your unique characteristics. These types are a basis for more specific treatment and should not be turned into stereotypes.

CONSTITUTION CHART

	VATA (AIR)	PITTA (FIRE)	KAPHA (WATER)
HEIGHT:	tall or very short	medium	usually short but can be tall and large
FRAME:	thin, bony	moderate, good muscles	large, well developed
WEIGHT:	low, hard to hold weight	moderate	heavy, hard to lose weight
SKIN LUSTER:	dull or dusky	ruddy, lustrous	white or pale
SKIN TEXTURE:	dry, rough, thin	warm, oily	cold, damp, thick
EYES:	small, nervous	piercing, easily inflamed	large, white
HAIR:	dry, thin	thin, oily	thick, oily, wavy, lustrous
TEETH:	crooked, poorly formed	moderate, bleeding gums	large, well formed
NAILS:	rough, brittle	soft, pink	soft, white
JOINTS:	stiff, crack easily	loose	firm, large
CIRCULATION:	poor, variable	good	moderate
APPETITE:	variable, nervous	high, excessive	moderate but constant
THIRST:	low, scanty	high	moderate
SWEATING:	scanty	profuse but not enduring	low to start but profuse
STOOL:	hard or dry	soft, loose	normal
URINATION:	scanty	profuse, yellow	moderate, clear

SENSITIVITIES:	cold, dryness, wind	heat, sunlight, fire	cold, damp
IMMUNE FUNCTION:	low, variable	moderate, sensitive to heat	high
DISEASE TENDENCY:	pain	fever, inflammation	congestion, edema
DISEASE TYPE:	nervous	blood, liver	mucous, lungs
ACTIVITY:	high, restless	moderate	low, moves slowly
ENDURANCE:	poor, easily exhausted	moderate but focused	high
SLEEP:	poor, disturbed	variable	excess
DREAMS:	frequent, disturbed	moderate, colorful	infrequent, romantic
MEMORY:	quick but absent-minded	sharp, clear	slow but steady
SPEECH:	fast, frequent	sharp, cutting	slow, melodious
TEMPERAMENT:	nervous, changeable	motivated	content, conservative
POSITIVE EMOTIONS:	adaptability	courage	love
NEGATIVE EMOTIONS:	fear	anger	attachment
FAITH:	variable, erratic	strong, determined	steady, slow to change

TOTAL	Vata_____	Pitta_____	Kapha_____

Prana, Tejas and Ojas

The Master Forms of Vata, Pitta and Kapha

Vata, Pitta and Kapha have subtle counterparts on the level of vital energy. These are Prana, Tejas and Ojas, which we will call the "three vital essences." Prana, Tejas and Ojas are the master forms of Vata, Pitta and Kapha. They control ordinary mind-body functions and keep us healthy and free of disease. If reoriented properly, they unfold higher evolutionary potentials as well. They are the positive essences of the three biological humors that sustain positive health. While increases in the biological humors promote disease, increases in the vital essences promote positive health (unless one of these is increased without properly developing the others). These three forces are the keys to vitality, clarity and endurance, necessary for us to really feel healthy, fearless and confident.

PRANA: primal life-force — the subtle energy of air as the master force behind all mind-body functions. It is responsible for coordination of breath, senses and mind. On an inner level, it governs the development of higher states of consciousness.

TEJAS: inner radiance — the subtle energy of fire through which we digest impressions and thoughts. On an inner level, it governs the development of higher perceptual capacities.

OJAS: primal vigor —the subtle energy of water as our vital energy reserve, the essence of digested food, impressions and thought. On an inner level it gives calm, and supports and nourishes all higher states of consciousness.

Psychological Functions of the Three Vital Essences

Prana in the mind allows it to move and respond to the challenges of life. Tejas in the mind enables it to perceive and to judge correctly. Ojas in the mind gives patience and endurance that provides psychological stability. Prana in our deeper consciousness energizes us throughout the process of reincarnation, giving life to all aspects of our nature. Tejas in consciousness holds the accumulated insight of our will and spiritual aspiration. Ojas in consciousness is the material power from which the soul produces all its various bodies.

Each of these three factors has an emotional effect as well. Prana maintains emotional harmony, balance, and creativity. Tejas gives courage, fearlessness, and vigor that allows us to accomplish extraordinary actions. Ojas provides peace, calm and contentment. Without these emotional sustaining forces, the mind cannot accomplish anything significant.

How Prana, Tejas and Ojas are Built Up

Prana, Tejas and Ojas are built up in two ways. On a gross level, they derive from the essence of the nutrients we take into the body as food, heat and air. On a subtle level, they are fed by the impressions we take in through the senses. Key to the functioning of Prana, Tejas and Ojas is the reproductive fluid, which functions as their container in the physical body. It is the ultimate product of the food we take in that holds our strongest energies.

Prana is the life-creating capacity inherent in the reproductive fluid. This creates children through the sexual act, but can be directed inwardly to rejuvenate both body and mind. Tejas is the capacity of the reproductive fluid to give courage and daring. For example, it enables male animals to fight with great strength in order to mate. Inwardly, it can give us vigor and decisiveness for any important action. Ojas is the power of the reproductive fluid to promote endurance, which provides the ability to sustain us not only sexually but through all forms of sustained exertion, physically and mentally. Without the proper reserve of reproductive fluids, we must be deficient in Prana, Tejas and Ojas, which can negatively impact both physical and psychological health. Ayurveda emphasizes preserving enough of our reproductive fluid to maintain these three vital essences. It also shows us ways to develop these three forces when they are insufficient.

On a subtle level, Ojas is fed through the sensory impressions of taste and smell. Tejas is the essence of the heat we absorb, not only through food but also through the skin, where we absorb sunlight. Tejas is fed through visual impressions. Prana is the vital energy we take in, not only through food but through liquids, and, of course, through breathing. Prana is carried by the fluids in our body, the blood and plasma, which serve as its vehicle. Our body fluids are energized by the Prana we take in. Prana is also absorbed through the senses of hearing and touch.[4]

Prana, Tejas and Ojas and Health Imbalances

Psychological imbalances are closely related to the conditions of Prana, Tejas and Ojas. Prana is responsible for the enthusiasm and expression in the psyche, without which we suffer from depression and mental stagnation. Tejas governs mental digestion and absorption, without which we lack clarity and determination. Ojas provides psychological stability and endurance, without which we experience anxiety and mental fatigue. Without the proper vital energies, the mind cannot function properly. We cannot heal the mind without improving and harmonizing its energies.[5]

We will refer to Prana, Tejas and Ojas as background concepts throughout the book. While not as important as Vata, Pitta and Kapha, they must not be overlooked either. Please relate them back to Vata, Pitta and Kapha as their positive forms, or to the elements of air, fire and water for easy understanding.

3. The Three Gunas: How to Balance Your Consciousness

We live in a magical universe filled with great forces of life and death, creation and destruction. Divine powers can be found everywhere to lift us into a greater peace and understanding. But "undivine" forces are also ever present, working to lure us down further into confusion and attachment. Truth and falsehood, ignorance and enlightenment form the light and dark, the illumination and shadow of the world. In this basic duality of creation, we struggle not merely to survive but also to find meaning in our lives. We must learn to navigate through these contrary currents so that we can benefit by the ascending spiritual force and avoid the descending unspiritual inertia.

Nature herself is the Divine Mother in manifestation and the universe is her play of consciousness. She provides not only for material growth and expansion that moves outward, but also supports our spiritual growth and development, which moves within. Nature possesses a qualitative energy through which we can either expand into wisdom or contract into ignorance. Nature functions through conscious forces, spirits if you will, which can be either enlightening or darkening, healing or harming. Most of these powers are unknown to us and we do not know how to use them. Trained as we are in a rational and scientific

manner to look to the outside, we lack the ability to perceive the subtle forces hidden in the world around us.
However, for any real healing of the mind to be possible,
we must understand these forces and learn how to work
with them as they exist, not only in the world but also in
our own psyche.

Ayurveda provides a special language for understanding
the primal forces of Nature and shows us how to work with
them on all levels. According to Yoga and Ayurveda,
Nature consists of three primal qualities, which are the
main powers of Cosmic Intelligence that determine our
spiritual growth. These are called gunas in Sanskrit, meaning "what binds," because wrongly understood they keep
us in bondage to the external world.

1) Sattva — intelligence, imparts balance
2) Rajas — energy, causes imbalance
3) Tamas — substance, creates inertia

The three gunas are the most subtle qualities of Nature
that underlie matter, life and mind. They are the energies
through which not only the surface mind, but also our
deeper consciousness functions. They are the powers of the
soul which hold the karmas and desires that propel us from
birth to birth. The gunas adhere in Nature herself as her
core potential for diversification.

All objects in the universe consist of various combinations of the three gunas. Cosmic evolution consists of their
mutual interaction and transformation. The three gunas
are one of the prime themes of Ayurvedic thought and will
occur throughout the book. They form a deeper level than
the three biological humors and help us understand our
mental and spiritual nature and how it functions.

SATTVA is the quality of intelligence, virtue and good-
ness, and creates harmony, balance and stability. It is light

(not heavy) and luminous in nature. It possesses an inward and upward motion and brings about the awakening of the soul. Sattva provides happiness and contentment of a lasting nature. It is the principle of clarity, wideness and peace, the force of love that unites all things together.

RAJAS is the quality of change, activity, and turbulence. It introduces a disequilibrium that upsets an existing balance. Rajas is motivated in its action, ever seeking a goal or an end that gives it power. It possesses outward motion and causes self-seeking action that leads to fragmentation and disintegration. While, in the short term, Rajas is stimulating and provides pleasure, owing to its unbalanced nature it quickly results in pain and suffering. It is the force of passion which causes distress and conflict.

TAMAS is the quality of dullness, darkness, and inertia and is heavy, veiling or obstructing in its action. It functions as the force of gravity that retards things and holds them in specific limited forms. It possesses a downward motion that causes decay and disintegration. Tamas brings about ignorance and delusion in the mind and promotes insensitivity, sleep and loss of awareness. It is the principle of materiality or unconsciousness that causes consciousness to become veiled.

CORRESPONDENCES OF THE THREE GUNAS

	SATTVA	RAJAS	TAMAS
Color	White purity & harmony	Red action & passion	Black darkness & delusion
Time	Day, clarity	Sunrise & Sunset twilight, transition	Night, darkness
Energy	Neutral or balanced	positive, sets things in motion	negative, retards motion
Worlds	heaven or space, the region peace	atmosphere the region of storms	earth, the realm the realm of of gravity and inertia
Levels of Cosmos	causal or ideal	subtle or astral, pure form	gross or physical
Kingdoms of Nature	spiritual beings: gods, goddesses and sages	human realm	mineral, plant & animal kingdoms
States of Consciousness	waking	dream	deep sleep

Sattva and the Mind

The mind, or consciousness in general, is naturally the domain of Sattva. Consciousness itself is called Sattva in Sanskrit. Unless the mind is calm and clear, we cannot perceive anything properly. Sattva creates clarity, through which we perceive the truth of things, and gives light, concentration and devotion. Rajas and Tamas are factors of mental disharmony, causing agitation and delusion. They result in wrong imagination and misperception.

From Rajas comes the false idea of the external world as real in itself, which causes us to seek happiness outside ourselves and lose track of our inner peace. Rajas creates desire, distortion, turbulence and emotional upset. It predominates in the sensory aspect of the mind because the senses are ever-moving and seeking various objects. As long as we remain immersed in the pursuit of sensory enjoyment, we fall under the instability of Rajas.

From Tamas comes the ignorance that veils our true nature and weakens our power of perception. Through it arises the idea of an ego or separate self, by which we feel ourselves to be alone and isolated. Tamas prevails in consciousness identified with the physical body, which is dull and limited. As long our identity and sense of well-being is primarily physical, we remain in the dark realm of Tamas.

Sattva is the balance of Rajas and Tamas, combining the energy of Rajas with the stability of Tamas. By increasing Sattva, one gains peace and harmony, and returns to Primordial Nature and Pure Spirit in which is liberation. However, attachment to Sattva, such as clinging to virtue, can bind the mind. For this reason we must strive to develop pure Sattva, which is its detached form, or Sattva not clinging to its own qualities. Pure Sattva does not condemn Rajas and Tamas, but understands their place in the cosmic harmony, which is as outer factors of life and body whose proper place is apart from our true nature.

When pure Sattva prevails in our consciousness, we transcend time and space and discover our eternal Self. The soul regains its basic purity and unites with God. When out of balance, the three gunas bring about the process of cosmic evolution through which the soul evolves through the kingdoms of Nature, experiencing birth and death, happiness and sorrow in various bodies. The movement of the three gunas is coterminous with creation.

Sattva as the state of balance is responsible for all true health and healing. Health is maintained by Sattvic living, which is living in harmony with Nature and our inner Self, cultivating purity, clarity and peace. Rajas and Tamas are the factors that cause disease. Rajas causes pain, agitation and the dissipation of energy. Tamas brings about stagnation, decay and death. Rajas and Tamas usually work together. Rajas brings about the over-expression of energy, which eventually leads to exhaustion, in which Tamas prevails.

For example, too much spicy food, alcohol, and sexual indulgence are initially Rajasic or stimulating. These eventually lead to such Tamasic conditions as fatigue and collapse of energy. On a psychological level, too much Rajas, which is turbulent emotion, leads to Tamas or mental dullness and depression.

Mental Types According to the Gunas

To have Sattva predominant in our nature is the key to health, creativity and spirituality. Sattvic people possess an harmonious and adaptable nature which gives the greatest freedom from disease, both physical and mental. They strive toward balance and have peace of mind that cuts off the psychological root of disease. They are considerate of others and take care of themselves. They see all life as a learning experience and look for the good in all things, even in disease, which they strive to understand, not merely to suppress.

Rajasic people have good energy but burn themselves out through excessive activity. Their minds are usually agitated and seldom at peace. They have strong opinions and seek power over others, often regardless of the means. They are impatient and inconsistent in dealing with their problems and do not wish to take the time or responsibility to get well. They blame others for their problems, including their therapists.

Rajasic people can accomplish their goals and are generally in control of their lives. However, they are not awake to their spiritual purpose, and are dominated by the ego in their pursuit of happiness. Life brings them shocks, which can cause them great suffering, particularly when they lose control. Even when they achieve their goals, they find that they are still not happy.

Tamasic types have deep-seated psychological blockages. Their energy and emotion tend to be stagnant and repressed, and they do not know what their problems really are. They do not seek proper treatment and usually have poor hygiene or poor self-care habits. They accept their condition as fate and do not take advantage of the methods that may alleviate their problems. They allow other people and negative influences to dominate them and do not like to be responsible for their lives. They prefer not to deal with their problems or will not let others know about them, which only allows the problems to get worse.[6]

Mental Constitution According to the Three Gunas

The gunas show our mental and spiritual state, through which we can measure our propensity for psychological problems. The following test is a good index of these qualities and how they work within our life and character.

The answers on the left indicate Sattva, in the middle Rajas, and on the right Tamas. Please fill out this form carefully and honestly. After answering the questionnaire for yourself, you should have someone who knows you well, like your husband, wife or close friend, fill it out for you also. Note the difference between how you view yourself and how others see you.

For most of us, our answers will generally fall in the middle or Rajasic area, which is the main spiritual state in our active and outgoing culture today. We will have various psychological problems but can usually deal with them. A Sattvic nature shows a spiritual disposition with few psychological issues. A highly Sattvic nature is rare at any time and shows a saint or a sage. A Tamasic person has a danger of severe psychological problems but would be unlikely to fill out such a chart or even read such a book. The areas in ourselves that we can improve from Tamas to Rajas or from Rajas to Sattva will aid in our peace of mind and spiritual growth. We should do all we can to make such changes.

MENTAL CONSTITUTION CHART

DIET:	Vegetarian	Some meat	Heavy meat diet
DRUGS, ALCOHOL & STIMULANTS:	Never	Occasionally	Frequently
SENSORY IMPRESSIONS:	Calm, pure	Mixed	Disturbed
NEED FOR SLEEP:	Little	Moderate	High
SEXUAL ACTIVITY:	Low	Moderate	High
CONTROL OF SENSES:	Good	Moderate	Weak
SPEECH:	Calm and peaceful	Agitated	Dull
CLEANLINESS:	High	Moderate	Low
WORK:	Selfless	For personal goals	Lazy
ANGER:	Rarely	Sometimes	Frequently
FEAR:	Rarely	Sometimes	Frequently
DESIRE:	Little	Some	Much
PRIDE:	Modest	Some Ego	Vain
DEPRESSION:	Never	Sometimes	Frequently
LOVE:	Universal	Personal	Lacking in love
VIOLENT BEHAVIOR:	Never	Sometimes	Frequently
ATTACHMENT TO MONEY:	Little	Some	A lot
CONTENTMENT:	Usually	Partly	Never
FORGIVENESS:	Forgives easily	With effort	Holds long-term grudges

CONCENTRATION:	Good	Moderate	Poor
MEMORY:	Good	Moderate	Poor
WILL POWER:	Strong	Variable	Weak
TRUTHFULNESS:	Always	Most of the time	Rarely
HONESTY:	Always	Most of the time	Rarely
PEACE OF MIND:	Generally	Partly	Rarely
CREATIVITY:	High	Moderate	Low
SPIRITUAL STUDY:	Daily	Occasionally	Never
MANTRA, PRAYER:	Daily	Occasionally	Never
MEDITATION:	Daily	Occasionally	Never
SERVICE:	Much	Some	None
Total:	Sattva_____	Rajas_____	Tamas_____

The Three Gunas and Therapy

Many different types of medical and healing therapies exist for the mind. To benefit from them properly and to avoid their possible side-effects, we must understand their approach and when they are useful. Here Ayurveda helps us greatly by showing how healing therapies relate to these three gunas. This provides us with a deep understanding of the healing process and its likely results. Sattvic therapies work through Sattvic qualities of love, peace and non-violence. Rajasic therapies work through Rajasic qualities of stimulation, energization and agitation. Tamasic therapies work through Tamasic qualities of sedation, sleep and grounding. Ayurvedic therapies are primarily Sattvic and employ Rajasic and Tamasic modalities only under special circumstances.

Sattvic healing uses Nature, the life force and the power of the cosmic mind, through such treatment methods as herbs, vegetarian diet, mantra and meditation. Rajas can occasionally be useful in the healing process. Rajas helps break up Tamas, while Sattva, being a condition of harmony, does not always have the ability to do so. It is often necessary to move from Tamas to Rajas in order to return to Sattva, like needing to stimulate or shock a person into awakening to their repressed pain. Tamas is seldom useful in the healing process except when required to sedate too high Rajas. For example, a person in hysteria, an excess Rajas condition, may require a strong sedative herb or drug, a Tamasic therapy. In this case Sattva would be too mild to calm Rajas.[7]

Ayurvedic psychology aims at moving the mind from Tamas to Rajas and eventually to Sattva. This means moving from an ignorant and physically-oriented life (Tamas), to one of vitality and self-expression (Rajas), and finally to one of peace and enlightenment (Sattva).[8]

Three Stages of Mental Healing

1) Breaking up Tamas/developing Rajas — moving from mental inertia to self-motivated action.

2) Calming Rajas/developing Sattva — moving from self-motivated action to selfless service.

3) Perfecting Sattva — moving from selfless service to meditation.

Naturally it is important to know what stage is appropriate for a person. A person in a Tamasic condition requires outer activity to break up their inertia; he or she cannot simply be asked to sit quietly and meditate. At such times Rajasic (active) methods are necessary and

Sattvic (passive) methods may not be sufficient. The person requires communication and working with other people. A person in a Rajasic condition, however, requires a reduction of activity and interiorization of consciousness (development of Sattva). Yet this must be done gradually because Rajas does not subside all at once. The person must be introduced into meditation through practical therapies of yogic postures, mantras or visualizations. A person in a Sattvic condition requires spiritual practices and not ordinary psychological treatment, and can easily move into meditation without much external support.

However, these three stages are not simply different levels. We all have Tamasic, Rajasic and Sattvic factors in our minds. We all need each of these three processes to some degree. There are times when our minds are Tamasic, like right after waking up in the morning or when daydreaming in the afternoon. Whenever we are mentally dull or emotionally depressed, Tamas is predominant. Rajas prevails when we are agitated, disturbed, active or outgoing, like when we are very busy working with a number of people or projects. Sattva prevails when we are quiet, peaceful and content, or naturally fall into meditation.

Similarly we should not judge other people by how they appear when dominated by one quality only. Even a spiritually advanced person has Tamasic moments or periods when he or she may do something regrettable. In the same way, spiritually undeveloped persons have Sattvic moments when they may do something inspired, noble or kind. When looking at ourselves, we should try to see all three factors in our nature and behavior and try to develop our Sattvic side.

Stage 1 — Personal Healing

Breaking Up Tamas/ Moving from Tamas to Rajas

For this transition, fire is necessary. We must wake up, act and begin to change. Deep-seated patterns of attachment, stagnation and depression must be released. We must recognize our suffering and learn from it, confronting our pain, including what we have suppressed or ignored for years. A new sense of who we are and what we need to do is required. Action (Rajas) is indicated, not only in the mind but involving outer aspects of our lives. We must break with the past, bring new energies into our lives, perhaps change jobs or modify our relationships, or move to a new locale.[9]

Stage 2 — Healing of Humanity

Calming Rajas/ Moving from Rajas to Sattva

For this transition, space is necessary. We must surrender our pain and give up our personal seeking, letting go of individual hurts and sorrows. Egoistic drives and motivations must be surrendered for the greater good. We must depersonalize our problems and look to understand the entire human condition and the pain of others. Leaving behind our personal problems, we must take up the problems of humanity, opening up to the suffering of others as our own. We must learn that life creates suffering in order to help us grow spiritually. This is a stage of service and charity.[10]

STAGE 3 — UNIVERSAL PEACE

Developing Pure Sattva

To bring about this transition, we must develop love and awareness as universal forces. We must learn to transcend the limitations of the human condition to our higher spiritual nature. Inner peace must become our dominant force. We should no longer seek to overcome our pain but to develop our joy. We should no longer be centered in our personal or collective problems but in developing communion with the greater universe and the Divine powers at work within it. At this stage we move from the human aspect of our condition to the universal aspect, becoming open to all life. This is the stage of spiritual practice. It is beyond all ordinary healing and works to heal our relationship with God or the inner Self.

As you go through this book remember the three gunas. We will explore how they work according to the different layers and functions of the mind. Go to the Sattvic core of your being to understand this wisdom of Ayurveda.

4. The Nature of the Mind

It is amazing to note that so many different ideas exist about the nature of the mind and how it functions. Different systems of psychology, philosophy and religion define the mind in ways that can be radically different or even contradictory to one another. All of us agree on the basic facts of the physical body — its form, structure and function. No one holds that the body has three legs, or that the stomach thinks and the brain digests food. The reason for this is that the body is easy to observe. Yet while we can easily list the main systems of the physical body, we find it difficult to do so for the mind. The mind appears as an amorphous or structureless entity, rather than a precise instrument like the body.

Though we all have minds and use them constantly, we do not know what our mind really is. We are so caught up in the mind's activities that we do not take the time to discover what the mind itself really is. In the realm of psychology, we are still groping in the dark, trying to treat an entity whose character eludes us. Without knowing the nature of the mind and its functions, how can we really approach it? After all, how we perceive the mind is the basis of any psychological diagnosis and treatment. The problem is that to know the mind we must first know ourselves. We must understand who we really are. Thought, as we ordinarily know it, is a function of the ego or separate self. A subjective personal bias colors how we look at the mind, rendering an objective assessment of its capacities almost impossible.

The first step in any true psychology, therefore, is to understand the mind and how it works. What is the nature of this marvelous instrument called the mind? What is its relationship with who we are? What is its connection with the body? What is the right function of the mind? Can we learn to see the mind as objectively as we see our hands and feet? Here Ayurveda and Yoga offer tremendous insights.

Getting to Know the Mind

Can one imagine being put into the driver's seat of an automobile with the engine running and not knowing how to drive, not knowing how to use the brakes, the steering wheel or the clutch? Naturally we would get into an accident and, should we survive, would end up permanently afraid of driving.

We are in a not too different situation with our minds. Our awareness is placed in the mind when we are born, but we are not taught how to use the mind, its sensitivities and emotions. We are not taught the meaning of its states of waking, dreaming, and deep sleep. We are not shown the comparative functions of reason, feeling, will and sensory perception. We are left in the dark because our parents and society do not understand the mind and how it works. The mind is the main vehicle we use for all that we do, yet few, if any of us, know how to use and care for it properly.

We all suffer from ignorance of the nature of the mind. All problems we encounter in life are based ultimately upon not knowing the mind and its functions. From this primary problem, various secondary problems arise — like how to fulfill our desires, or how to avoid what we fear — which, however important these may appear, are merely the natural consequence of this basic ignorance about the mind. For example, if we do not know how to drive a car properly, the issue of where to go with it is not important. However, we take these derivative problems as primary or blame others for them, turning them into social, moral, or political issues, not realizing, that they are just one problem — not understanding the mind. From a wrong understanding of the mind, we develop wrong ideas about the world and run into difficulty in our social interactions.

To use another analogy, if we do not understand how fire works, we may burn ourselves. This does not mean we are a bad person or that fire is bad, but only that we do not understand fire and its properties. The mind has its qualities and, like fire, can be used for both good and bad. It can provide great happiness or wreak tremendous havoc in the world, as history has shown again and again. All psychological problems are nothing more than a wrong use of the mind, which arises from ignorance of how the mind works. The solution to all our mental problems is to learn to use the mind properly. This is true whatever our psychological problems may be.

More important than any examination of our personal or social problems is educating ourselves about the nature of the mind. All the problems that appear so immediate and important — like whether we will be loved or if our friends and family can be happy — are not the real issue and cannot be solved directly. The real issue is how to use the most important and central instrument in our lives — the mind itself.

Learning the right use of the mind not only solves our psychological problems, but directs us to our higher potential of Self-realization. It leads to the spiritual life, which is our real occupation as conscious beings. Then we

can transcend the mind — which is inherently limited —
to Pure Awareness unbounded by time, space or causation.
For all things in life, we must start with understanding the
mind.

Mind as an Object

Though we have always had a mind, most of us have
never taken the time to observe it. Let us look at our
minds. For this we must step back internally and take the
role of the observer. We must begin to witness the mind
and its functions.[11] Imagine that your thoughts are a
stream and you are sitting on the bank watching them
flow by. Learn to see the contents of the mind flowing by,
without judgment or interference, just as you might
observe the currents or debris floating down a river.

By taking such a witnessing attitude, we can easily get
to know the mind and its activities. We can perceive various fluctuations in thoughts, feelings and impressions, and
various states of waking, dreaming and deep sleep. We
should strive to maintain our awareness in the attitude of
witnessing the mind. This is the key for learning what the
mind is. As long as we are caught up in the mind's activities, we cannot see the mind as it is, just as we cannot
observe what is going in a theater if our attention is
engrossed in the movie.

Whatever we can observe, like a cup upon the table, is
an object and exists apart from our awareness, which is its
perceiver. Yet we cannot only observe external objects, we
can also observe internal objects. We can note whether our
sense organs are acute or impaired, as when our vision
begins to fail. Similarly we can observe our emotions, our
thoughts, and even our own ego, which are all fluctuating
phenomena, if we look deeply. We can observe the func-

tions of the mind just as we can observe the movements of our body.

Just as the eye is not damaged when a cup falls onto the floor and breaks, so consciousness is not damaged when the contents of the mind get altered or damaged. The witnessing consciousness is apart from the objects and conditions that it observes. Therefore, the first thing we observe about the mind is that, as something observable, the mind is an object. The mind is material and part of the external world. It belongs to us but it is not who we really are, just as our house belongs to us but is not us. This may be shocking to consider, but it is really something intuitively known to us. When we speak of "my mind," we are defining the mind as an object that belongs to us and not as ourselves.

The mind has a material structure, a set of observable energies and conditions. This is not to say that the mind is a gross object like a stone or that it is an organ in the physical body like the brain, or that it is merely chemical in nature. The mind is not physical matter, but it is matter of a subtle nature, ethereal and luminous. As an organic entity, the mind has a structure, a cycle of nutrition, an origin and an end. The mind is invested with a certain quantum of energy that produces various tangible effects.

Just as we can both see and use our hands, so awareness can perceive and use the mind. But this requires a very high state of attention. It requires detachment from the mind, which means detachment from the mind's activities and interests.

Mind as an Instrument

The second important fact about the mind, which follows from the mind's material nature, is that the mind is an instrument or tool. The sense organs themselves are instruments — the eye an instrument of seeing, the ear an instrument of hearing, and so on. Similarly, the mind that works to process sensory information is itself an instrument. The mind is a means of deriving information from the external world. The mind is the main instrument we use to function in life. The mind is an instrumentality of knowing devised by Cosmic Intelligence to allow for consciousness to gain experience. The mind is the ultimate machine, the best computer, the highest organization of matter possible, which allows for the material world to be cognized.

Notice that we are speaking of the mind, not the brain. The brain is the physical organ through which the mind works. We are not conscious of the brain itself or its structure. We are only conscious of our actual thought process. The mind is not the brain, but is more subtle. The brain is the vehicle for the mind and mirrors its operations, but the mind is not limited to the physical apparatus of the brain, any more than a person is limited to his shadow.

Note that we speak of "my" mind, indicating that we view the mind like an instrument. We can direct our attention. We can employ our reasoning faculty. We can develop our will. We can cultivate our feelings. But if the mind is an instrument, then we are not the mind, just as we are not any other instrument we use in life. Like any instrument, we are the one who uses and must master it, not let it tell us what to do.

However, we have forgotten that the mind is our instrument, though we speak of the mind as ours and not of ourselves as the mind. We let the mind tell us who we are and what to do. Having become slaves of the mind, we lose control of our destiny and fall under the desires of the

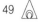

mind, which are not our own but come from the external world.

Awareness and the Mind

Behind changing mental fluctuations is a constant awareness, an unbroken sense of self or being, an ongoing ability to observe, witness and perceive.[12] Though the contents of the mind constantly shift, like clouds in the sky, there is an ongoing continuity to our consciousness, like the purity of space, through which we can observe these with detachment. Therefore the mind itself is not awareness. It is the instrument that awareness works through, like the computer a person works with.

Awareness, unlike the mind, has no form, function or movement. It is not located in time and space but stands apart as their witness. It is not affected by action and remains free of good and bad results. To know this awareness, we must learn to go beyond the mind, which means to disengage from its involvements. This is our real work as human beings and the essence of the spiritual path, whatever form of it we choose to follow. As long we are in the sphere of the mind, we are dominated by the external and cannot know the inner reality.

True awareness is Pure Consciousness beyond the mental field. Our ordinary awareness is conditioned within the mental field. Only because the light of pure awareness is reflected onto the mental field does the mind appear to be conscious. The mind itself, therefore, is not aware, intelligent or self-luminous. It works through the reflection of a greater light, a greater consciousness in which alone is understanding and freedom. We must learn to seek that pure light beyond the mind.

Mind-Body Unity

The mind is organically related to the physical body. We can observe this by noting how our mind's functions change with physical fluctuations, how our behavior changes along with our diet, exercise patterns or intake of sensory impressions. The mind is also a kind of body or organism. It has its metabolism, its appropriate food, its waste products, and its derangements that can occur from its malfunction. These we will explore in detail in the later chapters of the book.

The physical body is primarily an organ of perception and expression. It is structured mainly by our sense organs, which provide perception, like the eyes and ears, and the motor organs, like the voice and hands, through which we express ourselves. The body, we could say, is the gross form of the mind. The body exists to allow the mind to perceive and act. Yet, though the mind-body complex is an organic unity, the mind and body are not the same. The mind can function apart from body consciousness as in sleep, trance and after-death states.

The body is an object of perception for the mind, as when we observe our hands or watch our breathing process. Most of the time we are not very aware of our bodies themselves, but are aware of some action with which they are involved. We are conscious of the body primarily when we are in pain or otherwise dominated by a strong bodily sensation, like sexual pleasure. When we are talking, reading or working, we are only slightly aware of our physical functioning. We are rarely conscious of our internal organs, like the liver or heart, except when we are sick. We mainly perceive the surface of the body through the skin and senses. Therefore, we are in the body but we are not the body.

Our true awareness or pure consciousness, however, transcends both mind and body. It is inherently free of their problems and limitations. But to get to it requires that we detach ourselves from mind-body functions.

Location of the Mind

There is no particular place in the physical body where the mind can be said to be located. Wherever we direct our attention, there the mind already is. You can see this for yourself. Whatever you look at, whether internally or externally, the mind is with you. The mind is not in the brain. It is not in the eye or the hand. It moves with our awareness. It is not even limited to the body because it can observe the body as an object and use it as an instrument.

Generally, we think that the mind dwells in either the head or the heart. The head is the center for the outer mind that works through the senses. The heart is the center of the inner mind or feeling nature that transcends the senses. The brain is no more than a screen on which the energies of consciousness from the heart get reflected. Ayurveda regards the heart as the center of consciousness.[13] This is not the physical heart but the core of knowing deep inside ourselves. We should not confuse this center with a physical location. It pervades all our mental activity.

Atomic Nature of the Mind

Having discussed the basic nature of the mind, we can now examine more deeply its structure. Look at how your attention functions and moves. The most important thing we see about the mind's structure is that the mind is atomic or point-like in nature. The mind consists of various points of thought, feeling and sensation, following one another in rapid succession. Again, you can observe this for yourself. Sit quietly and see how your senses work, like looking at a tree. Note the shifting movement of your mind and how it tries to construct the reality of the object from its moving points of attention.

The mind has no particular shape or size. It assumes the shape and size of whatever object that we examine. Yet it always consists of a series of points of attention. The mind is not an atom existing in space but a point-sized awareness which precedes and transcends all other material components and interactions.

Though the mind is atomic in nature, it can pervade the body as a whole, just as a dot of sandalwood oil can pervade the entire body by its fragrance. In this way, the mind can not only focus on different parts of the body but can motivate it as a whole. Similarly, it can pervade our entire field of perception. Though this only lasts an instant, these instants follow one another, giving us a sense of an entire field of awareness.

The atomic nature of the mind leads to various limitations. We can only focus on one particular object at a time. Our awareness has the nature of a shifting point. This allows us to place our attention in specific directions. At the same time it gives the mind a tendency to become narrow and attach itself only to those points of view it has already seen. We do not see the whole, but try to construct it by putting together various points of view. This process limits us to a perspective, and however many perspectives we have, there is always something that we miss.

The mind is like a pointillist painter. It is constructing reality out of points. Yet the reality must ever elude it as one can never arrive at the whole through fragments. The mind's knowledge is inherently limited by the point-like nature of the mind. The mind gives a series of snapshots, which allows us to construct a view of reality. But its snap-shots distort that reality by presenting only one side of it.

As each mind is a mere point of awareness, each mind is unique, has its own perspective, and potentially its own inherent bias. Each one of us is true to the perspective of our minds. We often fail to see, however, that this per-spective is not universal or even common, but the expres-sion of limitation.

Mobile Nature of the Mind

Our ever-shifting mental panorama of thoughts, emo-tions and sensations reveals the constantly changing or mobile nature of the mind. The mind is extremely volatile and impossible to prevent from moving. This is because the mind is not only a shifting point in space, but is also a changing point in time. The mind is not only in motion, the mind is its motion. Without motion, the mind does not function.

Our stream of consciousness is nothing but a rapid series of point flashes of mental activity. In fact, the mind is the prime point from which the ideas of time and space are constructed. It is like the point of an artist's pen which draws lines to create a sense of perspective.

The mind consists of a series of mental actions, which are never the same, even for an instant. If we look deeply, we see that the mobility of the mind is not continuous like a stream of water or oil. It is like a series of lightning flash-es, discontinuous and occurring in rapid succession, which allows us to put together a continuous image. The mind, therefore, is impossible to still, though there is a stillness beyond the mind.

Subtle and Sensitive Nature of the Mind

Have you ever tried to control your mind? You quickly find that the mind is subtle in nature and unpredictable like the wind. It has force, energy and movement, but it does not have a particular form. Like the wind, we can observe the mind more easily through what it moves and affects, rather than see it directly. The mind, like the wind, blows the clouds of thoughts and feelings. Yet the mind is not only like the wind, it is also like space. It encompasses and pervades all its contents, like a screen that holds all the pictures placed upon it. The mind is the most subtle form of matter. This we will examine in more detail in the next chapter on the mind and the elements.

The mind is very sensitive. It is the very organ of sensitivity underlying all the senses. Everything affects or colors the mind. Everything that we see or feel leaves some imprint or residue upon it. Hence the mind must be treated with care, particularly in children. The mind can be easily hurt, in which case it places barriers around itself and dulls its sensitivity. The mind is easily affected and disturbed, excited, depressed or distracted.

The mind takes the form of the objects it perceives. Hence it is very difficult to see the mind. When our awareness has withdrawn from the senses, our minds remain filled with thoughts and feelings. Only when we empty the mind of thought can we see the mind and recognize its basic insubstantiality, like a screen that has no meaning apart from the images projected on it.

Dualistic Nature of the Mind

The mind, like all matter, is dualistic in nature. It consists of opposite forces in various degrees of interaction. It is prone to dualistic reactions of like/dislike, love/hate and so on. Whatever we think about also creates its opposite. To assert one thing, we must also suggest the contrary.

This is why it is important not to train the mind with negativity, sin and guilt. For example, if we tell a person not to think of a monkey, he or she will naturally think of a monkey. If we tell a person not to do something, we have first asked them to think about doing it. If we assert the thought that we are happy, it suggests the idea that we are sad. Thought always reinforces its opposite.

The mind moves between opposites and is prone to ambivalence or extremes. It can easily become caught in opposites or become the victim of its own tendency to reverse itself. For this reason we should not try to force the mind in any particular direction, but seek to calm it from any extremes.

Difficulty in Controlling the Mind

Because of its volatile, point-like, subtle and dualistic nature, the mind is hard to grasp and almost impossible to control. It has a nature and movement of its own, which it tends to impress upon us or make us vulnerable to. Indeed, there is nothing more difficult to control than the mind. Human life is nothing but a struggle to learn to control the mind. If we have accomplished this, we have done everything and accomplished the most difficult thing in the entire universe. Inability to control the mind causes sorrow and is behind the disease process.

Mind and Thought

The mind is nothing but thought, which is the process of the mind. The mind is the entity made up by our thoughts. Take away the thoughts of the mind and the mind will disappear. As are our thoughts, so moves our mind, and so we become. Thought forms are also material and affect us like small, almost imperceptible, point-like electrical shocks. Our minds are constantly giving out and taking in thought forms, which either elevate or depress it. As we become more aware, we learn to consciously project positive thought forms and avoid those which are negative. Much of healing consists of changing the thought forms that dominate our lives. We must learn to project thoughts of peace, love, and harmony to counter those of conflict, unhappiness and disturbance that weaken our physical and mental vitality.

However, thought is of many types and occurs on many layers. Only if we change our deepest thoughts can we really change ourselves and get beyond the limitations of the mind. This is much more than changing our ideas about things; it means altering our deepest feelings and instincts. It requires deep prayer and meditation, profoundly energized and concentrated higher thought forms to counter deep-seated habits and addictions.

A Practical Experiment with the Mind

Examine for yourself the nature of your mind. Take an object, preferably one in the natural world, like a tree. Direct your attention to it. Note how your attention changes from instant to instant as you attempt to observe it. Note how, through a series of shifting perceptions, you construct the idea or total form of the tree, which you never perceive all at once. Try to hold your attention on one point of the tree. Notice how your attention cannot be held in one place but constantly moves around of its own accord.

As a further experiment, examine your emotions. See how your mind functions when you are angry or sad. Note the changing nature of emotions, how the stronger the emotion, the shorter it is likely to last. See how closely like and dislike, love and hate are bound together, and how emotions fluctuate like waves on the sea.

Next look at your thoughts. See how one thought follows another in rapid succession in a compulsive and erratic flow. Examine the habits of your thinking pattern. Note that much of what you think about has little practical value, but is merely the mind moving obsessively in its own memory grooves.

Finally examine the ego or "I-thought." See how this is the root of the other thoughts and how the mind is basically self-enclosed in its function. Try not to think the thought "I." See that this is not possible. The "I" is the inherent referential point, the center of the mind.

Learn to use your mind like a tool, develop various such experiments or observations, and, in this way, you will cease to be the victim of this subtle instrument. Once we learn to observe the mind, we will cease to be the victims of what goes on in our minds. Gaining control of our minds, we will no longer be dominated by the impulses coming from the senses and the conditioning of the external world. We will be able to be who we really are and create what is in harmony with the aspirations of our hearts.

5. The Five Elements and the Mind

Have you ever looked at the workings of your mind the way you would observe the world of Nature around you? According to Ayurveda, if we want to understand how our mind works, the best way is to look at how Nature operates. We must see how wind, fire and rain function in the psyche. We must learn to observe the storms of emotion, the light or half-light of reason, and all the rhythms through which not only our body, but also our mind and senses move. The mind is a formation of Nature, created according to her marvelous organic intelligence. The mind has the same basic structure as the universe and follows the same immutable laws. We live in a multi-level cosmos, including matter, energy, and mind on parallel and interdependent levels, like a magnificent crystal or gigantic lotus. Each level helps us understand the others and, through the outer, we gain the key to the inner.

The five elements are one of the main themes of Ayurvedic thought, and of related spiritual and healing systems. They are a great analog for all existence. Most of us do not think of the mind in terms of the elements, however. Yet, as a part of Nature, the mind also reflects the great elements through which Nature functions. To introduce the Ayurvedic view of the mind, we can approach it according to the elements.

Mind and the Elements

The mind transcends all the five gross elements because, through the mind, we can perceive all the elements and their interrelationships. We can observe, imagine and contemplate all the forms of earth, water, fire, air and ether. Yet the elements do provide a key to how the mind works. Though the elements in the mind are more subtle than those in the body, they retain the same basic attributes and actions. We can understand the mental elements through the analogy of the physical.

The mind is a creation primarily of the ether element of Nature. In substance, the mind is like space — expansive, open and all-pervading. Like space, it can hold innumerable forms and not be exhausted by them. The more evolved the mind becomes, the greater becomes its space. The less evolved the mind, the less expansive its space. Sorrow is nothing but a constricted mind space, like a bird in a cage. Bliss is an unlimited mind space, like a bird flying free in the sky.

In movement, however, the mind is like the wind. Air is its secondary element. There is nothing faster in movement than the mind. It is faster even than the speed of light. Look at your mind. It is always busy coordinating the body and senses, gathering information, making judgments, reacting emotionally, and endlessly thinking. This ongoing movement occurs because of the mind's connection with the air element.

Though ether and air are the main elements relating to the mind, the other elements have their place in the mind as well. The mind has its fire or light through which it can perceive things. This gives the mind a quality of illumination and a capacity of understanding. Similarly, the mind has a watery quality of emotion, empathy and feeling.

Finally, it carries a certain weight of earth, memory, and attachment. The mind contains all the elements within itself according to its differing qualities and actions.

The most subtle aspect of the elements makes up the mind. The mind space is more subtle than the physical space, which it pervades. The mind's air-like movement travels even in front of the wind. Fire in the mind can even perceive all external forms of light. Water in the mind or emotion is more subtle even than the external air. Earth in the mind, the mind's weight of attachments and opinions, cannot be weighed. The causal or seed level of the elements makes up the mind and through it create the gross or physical elements.

The Three Layers of the Mind

The mind has three basic layers — inner, intermediate and outer.

1) The inner mind consists of the deep core of feeling and knowing. It holds the tendencies that we carry deep inside ourselves and may never express or come to grips with in our outer lives.

2) The outer mind is the part of the mind dominated by the senses and emotions in which we ordinarily function on a daily basis, gathering impressions and acting in the outer world.

3) The intermediate mind is our capacity to bring outer impressions to the inside and inner tendencies to the outside. It mediates between transient sensory impressions and emotions on one side, and deep and abiding internal feelings on the other. It functions through reason and

perception to help us make judgments and
decisions.

These three aspects of the mind follow a similar model
as Vata, Pitta and Kapha or air, fire and water, taking this
energetic to a deeper level.

Inner Mind or Deeper Consciousness — Air

Air exists in the mind as the underlying mental sensitivity or deeper feeling nature. It is the background vibratory field of energies, habits and tendencies that sustain
the mind, by which we are continually thinking. Air is the
capacity of the mind to relate, identify itself and feel alive.
Through it we move, act and function as conscious beings.
It constitutes the heart or core consciousness, which is not
always evident at the surface but is the motivating force
behind the mind's other functions.

Like air, the mind possesses a capacity for change,
response, and transformation, and consists of various energies and impulses in a self-adjusting field. Our consciousness is a field of motion, an interacting dynamism of tendencies, latencies and impressions, only a few of which
reach the outer or self-conscious mind which dominates
our normal waking state. Most of what we call the unconscious, subconscious and superconscious is this inner
mind, of which we are not ordinarily aware.

This vibratory field of core thoughts and feelings, however, is a conditioned consciousness. It constitutes the
spontaneous and automatic habits and tendencies within
us. It is different from pure or unconditioned consciousness which is our true Self (note below).

Intermediate Mind or Intelligence — Fire

Fire exists in the mind as the rational or discriminating

faculty which allows us to perceive and to judge things. Our determinations of what is true and false, real and unreal, good and bad, valuable or worthless are outcomes of this capacity to weigh, measure and evaluate. It allows us to examine impressions to discern the object from our impression of it. It enables us to judge our experience to discover what it really means. In this way, it mediates between the inner core consciousness and our outer sensory functions.

Reason, like fire, has a hot and luminous nature that provides the ability to ascertain and discern. Reason, like fire, burns, digests and converts things into more subtle forms that nourish our awareness. Reason digests our impressions, feelings and thoughts and allows us to derive knowledge from them, putting each in its appropriate place relative to our understanding of reality.

Intelligence is the part of our consciousness articulated rationally and, therefore, brought to light. The greater and unarticulated part of the mind, the deeper consciousness, remains unconscious to our ordinary mind, and therefore appears to be dark. We enter into the rational part of the mind for important judgments, decisions and to arrive at real understanding. It is the part of the greater field of consciousness that we have brought to light and made our own.

Outer Mind, Sensation-Emotion — Water

Water exists in the mind as the emotional nature, our ability to connect with the external world, which is the seeking of consciousness to take form. This includes our capacity to gather sensory impressions and respond to them through like and dislike, attraction and repulsion, fear and desire.

Water is the formative aspect of mind which allows us to imagine, plan and construct our reality. It is the basis of will, motivation and action in the external world. It is the part of the mind, ever flowing outward, seeking to incarnate itself in matter and accumulate for itself the things of the world. Similarly, it is ever gathering impressions from the outside, allowing us to hold and accumulate them within.

Through the outer mind and its expressive capacity, we function in the world and feel ourselves to be part of an outer reality. It is what we usually know of as the mind and contains our ordinary thoughts, emotions and sensations.

The Two Levels of the Self

There are two basic levels to the self, between which the three aspects of consciousness function. The outer self defines itself according to the body, our physical identity. On the other side, the inner self is our sense of pure subjectivity, the pure "I am" beyond all bodily identity. These can be understood according to the model of earth and ether.

Outer Self, Ego — Earth

Earth exists in the mind as the ego, the sense of separate self through which we feel ourselves to be a limited person, identified with a particular body in time and space. Ego connects us to the physical body and allows us to discharge its functions as if they were our own. It provides a sense of self in the world, so that we can act within it.

The ego provides an objective referent or identity for the self. It works through a self-image or subject-object combination. It is the self in process, in becoming and is always seeking acquisition or achievement. Through ego-consciousness, we are ever trying to become somebody or get something in the outer world. It is consciousness objectified.

Inner Self, Soul — Ether

Ether exists in the mind as its underlying mind-space, the background capacity for all mental functions, vibrations and impressions. Without space, the mind cannot function and has no room to move. But like the external space, we seldom are aware of this internal mind-space. We enter it when we learn to be detached and not identify with the activities of the mind. From it we can observe the mind and transcend its limited patterns, which are like clouds in this higher mind-space.

Reflected in this mind-ether, we discover our higher identity as a soul, a conscious perceiver who transcends any body, image or identity. The inner self is a pure subjectivity, the pure "I am" or "I am that I am," as opposed to the "I am this" or "this is mine," the self-image which constitutes the ego. The inner self is content in its self-worth and finds peace in its own identity. It does not need to seek anything in the external world, which appears like a shadow before it.

Just as the ego or outer self separates us from other creatures, the soul or inner self unites us with them. As the ego possesses the vision of difference, the soul has the vision of unity. As the ego grasps form, the soul discerns the essence. Yet the individual Self or soul is still linked with the mind-body complex and its conditioning. In its pure form, divested of attachment to the mind, it becomes the Universal Self that transcends any individual identity and is beyond all manifestation. This is the unification of the individual with the universal Self in which there is liberation and immortality. This higher Self is the pure or unconditioned consciousness beyond the different levels of the mind.

Five Levels of the Mind

Ether — Higher Self
Air — Inner Consciousness
Fire — Intelligence
Water — Sense Mind
Earth — Ego

Workings of the Levels of the Mind

The outer mind is the doorway by which impressions from the external world enter into our consciousness through the gates of the senses. Intelligence, or intermediate mind, is the doorman who determines which impressions and energies can come in. Consciousness, or the inner mind, is the interior of the room in which these energies get deposited in the form of memories and tendencies, after they are allowed to enter.

Once impressions have become deposited in our inner consciousness, they grow like seeds and eventually impel us to act according to their nature. They produce various motivations, which result in the actions or karmas that determine the movement of our lives.

Impressions do not automatically enter into the inner mind. They only come in when we react to things in the form of dualistic emotions, likes and dislikes, love and hate, acceptance and rejection. Mere sensory perception by itself does not cause external energies to enter the mind. Detached observation cuts off external forces from entering the mind, while allowing us to observe them for what they are and respond to them appropriately. Detached observation digests impressions, allowing us to learn from them and not be limited by them.

As the doorkeeper, intelligence has the capacity to control the outer or sense mind and determine what comes in. This depends upon the principles according to which our reason is trained to work. If our reasoning faculty is not clear, then we rationalize our likes and dislikes rather than discern the truth of things. Reason, like a doorkeeper who has been bribed, lets any influence into the mind and then seeks a reason to justify letting it stay.

Our inner mind, the deeper feeling nature of the heart, is passive and innocent like a child. Whatever we open up our heart to gets deposited within it. The feeling nature is sensitive and vulnerable. It can be disturbed or motivated by whatever we let in. Therefore, it is very important to discriminate properly what we let into our hearts. Once we have accepted things at a heart level, we regard them as our own and can no longer examine them objectively, just as a mother can never criticize her own children.

The Perceptual Process

Let us examine our perceptual process to clarify this further. First we gather impressions based upon where we place our attention. For example, we look out the window and see the stature and dress of a person walking by. This is the function of the outer mind. Second we evaluate the impressions and come to a conclusion about what the object is. It is our neighbor, Sam. This is the function of intelligence. Third, the impression of the object gets deposited in our deeper consciousness as a memory. We remember that Sam walked by the house this morning. In this process ego surfaces at some point, generally after recognizing the object.

When we recognize our neighbor, we remember that we like him for some remark he said about us.

The outer mind works to select and gather impressions. It provides images like an object seen in a mirror, which is merely presented but not perceived. Intelligence, or the intermediate mind, allows us to recognize particular objects from the field of impressions. The ego allows us to identify an impression as belonging to us or to otherwise subjectively react to it. The inner mind, or feeling nature, allows the impression to be deposited and causes us to hold a feeling about it.

Action

The outer or sense mind allows us to act. It is the instrument through which ideas get transmitted to the motor organs. Through our intelligence, we are able to know what we are doing. It determines the idea, purpose or goal behind our action. Through the ego, we are able to identify with what we are doing as "I am doing this" or "I am doing that." Through the inner mind, we are able to feel the effects of what we are doing inside ourselves as long-term happiness or sorrow.

Our intentionality — what we want to do — which reason determines, decides the sensory impressions to which we are open. In this way, action and perception always go together. There are any number of impressions occurring at any given moment, but we can only register those which relate to what we regard as important. According to our plans and actions, we are always in motion in a particular direction, like a man driving a car. We must notice and give importance mainly to the impressions along the road that we have chosen to travel.

Levels of Awareness

Ego, or outer self, is the capacity to identify our consciousness with external objects and conditions. Ego is always bringing external impressions into the mind and making us feel dependent upon them. It tells us "I am this" or "this is mine." Through this, it makes us dependent upon external things for our identity and happiness. We rarely develop an awareness of the underlying mind-space or inner Self unless we learn the art of self-observation through meditation. Then we can discriminate who we are from external identities, actions and involvement.

What we normally call thought is the movement of the outer or sense mind in its planning and calculating capacity. Such thoughts are "I want to do this, tomorrow I should do that," and other activities of the ego. Emotion is also usually a movement of the sensate mind, an "I want to have this" (desire), or "I don't want to experience that" (fear). It is our emotional reactions to things, which are triggered by sensory impulses.

Intelligence functions when we attempt to determine what is true, good, of lasting value or of deep meaning. It also functions whenever we have to identify objects in the external world. The heart or consciousness is the home of our deep-seated states of mind, our enduring feelings, or the essence of our experience. We come into this only when we feel deeply, as in the peak and crisis experiences of our lives.

Normally all five functions are mixed up, confused by the rule of the ego, and we are unable to discern properly between them. The ego colors our reason and distorts our intelligence. It motivates the sense-mind to seek things in the external world. It casts a shadow over the heart and narrows our sense of feeling around its limited identities.

Usually our consciousness resides in the outer mind, lit up as it is by the lights of the senses. Because of the over-whelming abundance of sensory impulses we have to deal with, it is very hard not to get caught in them. Only when we are contemplating, reasoning or thinking deeply do we truly enter into the intermediate mind or intelligence. Only when we feel things deeply, and particularly in deep sleep and death when we withdraw from the realm of the senses, do we really come into the inner mind.

The inner mind is a dark realm for us because our atten-tion is externally directed through the outer mind. Only if we withdraw from our involvement in the external world of the senses can the inner world or realm of the inner mind become illumined. Then, when we close our eyes, we will see not darkness but light. True psychology is con-cerned with illumining this inner world. The inner mind is the dark interior, which is mainly unconscious for us and which, like a dark realm, tends to breed negative condi-tions and to store what we wish to avoid.

Unless we learn to look within, we will remain trapped in the outer mind and not know how to penetrate through the core of ignorance within us. The idea of the outer self or ego keeps our consciousness trapped in the outer mind. Only in contact with our inner Self can we unlock the secrets of awareness.

Psychological Problems and the Energetics of the Mind

As long as the elements in our consciousness are out of balance, the mind must be disturbed. The imbalance of energies of the mind, like that of the biological humors in the body, must produce disease or unrest.

The mind's true nature is subtle and must be purified

of the gross elements, particularly the earth element which accumulates through the ego. Consciousness and inner Self are of the nature of air and space. As long as we are caught in the heavier and lower functions of the mind, its true nature cannot be revealed. This is not just an issue of balancing the forces in the mind, but of spiritualizing the mind. We must reduce the lower functions and open up the higher. We must form an outer sensory orientation to an inner spiritual awareness.

Our psychological problems develop in the outer mind as we try to find happiness as a physical creature or ego-self. They leave memories like scars in the inner mind, just as a disease starts with external factors like bad diet or exposure to pathogens and gradually comes to affect our deeper organs and tissues. To heal the mind, we must purify the mind and the substances that compose it. To do this we must understand our consciousness and its functions. Now we will look at each of these separately. For this we will build on this energetic basis, placing this understanding of the elements into the background.

The Five Bodies

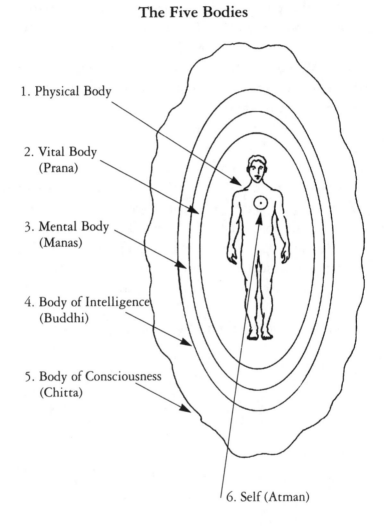

1. Physical Body

2. Vital Body
   (Prana)

3. Mental Body
   (Manas)

4. Body of Intelligence
   (Buddhi)

5. Body of Consciousness
   (Chitta)

6. Self (Atman)

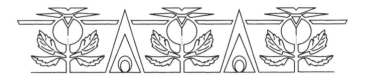

Part II

THE ENERGETICS OF CONSCIOUSNESS

Having gained an Ayurvedic perspective on the mind and body, now we are prepared to examine in depth the Ayurvedic view of consciousness and its functions. Yoga and Ayurveda divide the mental field into consciousness, intelligence, mind, and self and explain each along with their interactions. We will explain how to understand these different aspects of the mind in our own life and behavior.

This information follows from and builds upon that of the previous section relative to the elements, gunas, and biological humors and their action on the mind. In this way, we will probe deeply into who we are and all the main issues of our existence, from the subconscious to the superconscious and beyond. The profundity of the Vedic understanding of both the mind and universe should become clear and help us move into the deeper levels of our own awareness.

The reader should recognize that this material may not be understood quickly or easily, and some time may be necessary to assimilate it. Understanding our consciousness is not just a matter of reading, but of deep thought and meditation.

6. Conditioned Consciousness: The Greater Mental Field

Summary

In this chapter we will refer to the inner mind as "consciousness" because it is a deeper level of awareness than our ordinary thoughts. However, as previously indicated, it is a "conditioned consciousness," bound within the field of space and time, not pure or unconditioned consciousness that is timeless and infinite. Unconditioned consciousness is our true Self, beyond all the movements of the mind. Conditioned consciousness consists of thought on all levels — conscious, unconscious or superconscious. Unconditioned consciousness consists of thought-free awareness beyond all ideas, emotions and sensations, however subtle or vast.

The entire movement of spiritual growth consists of shifting from conditioned to unconditioned consciousness. Conditioned consciousness is the storehouse of all memories and attachments, from which psychological problems must ever arise. This conditioning of the mind distorts our perception and disturbs our emotions. Ayurvedic psychology works to calm the conditioned mind, removing its negative patterns that lead to disease and sorrow. However, the conditioned mind is not merely personal, but connects to all conditioned consciousness, all thought that exists within the universe, and the minds of all beings. We

cannot examine our own mind without looking at the
whole of life.

Consciousness — the World Within

What is consciousness? Through what do we think, feel
and perceive? How is it that we can be aware of anything?
While these are easy questions to pose, they are very difficult to answer. The way to examine them is to begin to
look into our consciousness and how it functions. Consciousness is the most wonderful thing in the universe.
There is no limit to its depth or to its grasp. It is like a vast
ocean but, unless we know how to navigate properly
through it, we can get lost. If we dive into it without the
right preparation, we can drown. Many mentally disturbed
people are so immersed in their internal consciousness that
they can no longer function in the external world. To us
they appear caught in delusion; in fact, they may be access-
ing deeper realities, although not in a wholesome manner.

Consciousness is our inner world. When the yogi looks
within he sees his consciousness pulsating with cosmic
forces; when we look within, however, we see only darkness or vague memories. Our external vision blinds us. We
are so conditioned to the vivid light of the senses that we
cannot perceive the subtle light of consciousness. Learning
to observe the contents of our consciousness is the most
important part of mental and spiritual development.
Ayurveda provides specific disciplines and meditation
techniques for this purpose. When consciousness is illumined, we transcend all external limitations. We no longer
need to experience the external world, because we have
learned its lesson — that all is within.

In Sanskrit, the greater mental field, or field of
thought, is called Chitta, from the root "chit," meaning

"to be aware." Chitta refers to the greater mind: unconscious, subconscious, self-conscious, and superconscious.[14]
Chitta is the mind or consciousness in general, the field
created by our thoughts. It specifically refers to the internal core of the mind, our center of pure feeling and direct
knowing. Chitta is the inner mind of which our outer or
personal mentality is a limited development. Out of con-
venience, I have translated Chitta as "consciousness," but
we should not forget that this is only an approximation.
Most of Chitta is unconscious to the ordinary mind. Only
in a spiritually developed person is the field of consciousness fully conscious or aware. Such a person can look at the
entire mental field because he or she has reached the pure
consciousness or Self beyond the limitations of thought.

What modern psychology calls the unconscious is but a
corner of this greater consciousness or Chitta. Modern psychology has penetrated into the personal unconscious and,
to some extent, the collective unconscious. Our potential
field of consciousness extends to all consciousness in the
universe, both individual and collective, personal and
impersonal, including God. It goes beyond all conditioned
consciousness to pure consciousness, which is the Absolute
or supreme truth. This is the field of yogic psychology
which is the psychology of the higher Self.

Chitta, the Body of Consciousness

Chitta is our core consciousness — the internal ground
of the mind. Consciousness, or the field of thought, is a
quickly vibrating subtle energy field, which is the basis of
all material manifestation. Chitta, as the core of the mind,
is the basic stuff or substance of consciousness. It constitutes the body or bulk of consciousness, just as the tissues
form the main substance of the physical body. The mind

and senses are like its arms and legs, its limbs and organs.

The physical body consists mainly of the heavy elements of water and earth and is a creation of gravity, which moves downward. Consciousness, on the other hand, is composed of the lighter elements of ether and air, and is a creation of our thoughts, which like a vapor move upward. While the heavy matters of our nature descend to the form of the physical body, the essence of our experience ascends to form our consciousness. We have a gross or gravity body (the physical) and a refined or essence body (consciousness).

We are not usually aware of our internal organs and tissues of the physical body, which are beyond the field of the senses. Similarly, we are seldom aware of our greater internal consciousness, which is not revealed by the outer functions of the mind. Our internal bodily processes function automatically, apart from our ordinary awareness. In the same way, our deeper consciousness maintains its process on a level deeper than the outer mind. However, we can become aware of this deeper consciousness. Meditation awakens us to its higher potentials.

Nature of Chitta

The nature of our core consciousness (Chitta) is sensitivity of all types, the capacity to feel in any manner. The ability to feel underlies all mental functions and develops into specific operations of thought, emotion and sensation. All that our minds do is a kind of feeling. Even reason is a kind of feeling, sensing or comparing. Such feeling is every response of our consciousness to stimuli, external or internal.

Consciousness is the capacity to relate, without which no feeling is possible. It allows us to feel things in ourselves and to feel ourselves in things. Our consciousness is a product of our deepest relationships, which determine how we feel about life. Association is a key factor determining the nature of our consciousness.

Consciousness registers everything that comes into the mental field on a level deeper than the outer mind. Without first being able to note things, other mental operations are not possible. Hypnosis can bring our awareness to the level of this deeper consciousness in which we can remember everything that has ever happened to us. Our deeper consciousness holds the memories of all that we experience, not only from birth but from previous lives. It carries the seeds that keep us involved in the cycle of rebirth, which are nothing but our deepest thoughts and impressions.[15]

Consciousness in the Natural World

The world comes into being through consciousness. Pure Consciousness is the unborn or Absolute beyond creation. Conditioned consciousness or thought (Chitta) is the ground of Nature, the primal substance that creates the universe. Consciousness is the substratum of everything, the first thing created that creates everything else. It is the essence of all possible experience. Thought creates everything, but this is a deeper and more primal level of thought than our ordinary personal reactions.

Consciousness is responsible for the existence and movement of the cosmos. It functions behind all forms of matter and energy. Some type of consciousness exists everywhere in Nature, even in inanimate objects. It sustains the cosmic process on all levels, starting with the atom itself. Whatever exists must contain some degree of consciousness or it could not be perceived. We are surrounded by the ocean of consciousness in which all things exist. Only part of it is individualized in the form of living creatures. The greater field of Cosmic Consciousness underlies the universe, animate and inanimate. Individual consciousness occurs within it as particularized centers, like waves on the sea.

Consciousness exists on a species level and holds the accumulated knowledge and experience of each type of creature. There are different types of consciousness relative to collective divisions of nation, sex, race, and religion, holding the specific tendencies of each group. As primal sensitivity, consciousness governs the plant kingdom, which lives in a state of deep sleep prior to the differentiation of the senses. Consciousness exists in a latent form in the elemental kingdom prior to the development of the life-force. It is the basis of the genetic code, which is its imprint on the cells, and governs core instinctual responses. A secret consciousness is working everywhere and is the key to all growth and development.

Consciousness becomes fully activated in angelic and divine beings, the denizens of the great formless heavens, where thought is the only reality. Consciousness embraces us both from the unconscious and the superconscious. On a subliminal level, a secret consciousness sustains our autonomic functions and works during sleep. On a superconscious level, a secret consciousness keeps track of our karma and supports our spiritual life.

The Superconscious

Our deeper consciousness contains the higher levels of the mind in which we can contact God and our inner Self. In it we retain knowledge of worlds more subtle than the physical. Consciousness extends beyond all realms of form into the realms of pure feeling and clear awareness.

Our individual consciousness links us to the collective consciousness, through which we can access the memories and tendencies of all human beings. This in turn links us with Cosmic Consciousness, through which we can access the experiences of all beings from minerals to gods. At the summit of the Cosmic Consciousness we contact God, the Divine Father/Mother, the cosmic Creator, Preserver and Destroyer.

Consciousness contains all knowledge, from the most mundane mechanics of the elements to the highest spiritual wisdom. Consciousness itself is the instrument of all internal forms of knowledge, transcending all knowledge gained by the senses. Awakening to the wisdom inherent in our deeper consciousness reveals to us all the mysteries of the universe. Consciousness is the source of true genius and insight. Gaining direct access to our deeper consciousness, we go beyond all external instruments of knowledge which, compared to its direct knowledge, are uncertain and vague.

However, thought-based consciousness (Chitta) is not the ultimate even in its cosmic dimensions. It is still a type of matter and not the pure immaterial Spirit. Beyond conditioned consciousness, both individual and cosmic, resides the Supreme Self, or Pure Consciousness. Unconditioned consciousness is called Chit in Sanskrit, compared to which conditioned consciousnesses (Chitta), including that of the Creator, are but reflections.[16]

The goal of life is not merely to explore the contents of consciousness but to dissolve them for the realization of the Self or Pure Consciousness beyond. All material objects, from a stone to Chitta itself, are external to our true nature. We must detach ourselves from them in order

to realize the truth. Only a purified consciousness, cleared
of its ego tendencies, has the power to bring about this
realization, which is the ultimate goal of all spiritual practice. Yet, even for ordinary mental health, we must have
some sense of our deeper nature beyond the fluctuations of
thought and emotion, which are inherently unstable.

Heart and Soul

Chitta also means the heart and dwells in the heart.
This is not the physical heart but the central core of deep
feeling and profound knowing, the spiritual heart. The
spiritual heart is contacted on the right side of the physical heart. In this regard Ayurveda differs from modern
medicine, which places the seat of consciousness in the
brain. According to Ayurveda, only our outer consciousness is situated in the brain, not our source awareness
which rests within the heart. Chitta is the psyche, or our
deeper mind, which is generally associated with the heart.

Chitta is the most intimate and enduring part of our
being. It is the mind of the soul, the individualized portion of Divinity that we are. The individual Self is the
reflection of the Supreme or Divine Self upon it. Our deeper consciousness holds our deepest aspiration, love and creativity, the peak experiences of life. In conditions of
extreme happiness, our consciousness gets immersed into
its internal core in which we forget all ordinary worries
and sorrows. We are all seeking to return to the peaceful
core of consciousness, which is to return to the heart. As
we move into our deeper consciousness, our heart opens
and our awareness expands into the Infinite. The calm and
clear heart reflects the Absolute and gives liberation from
the cycle of rebirth.

Our deeper consciousness is the level at which traumas

most affect us and where they get deposited deep inside us, particularly the sufferings of birth and death. There we hold our deeper sorrows, attachments, fears and anxieties. We must get to this level to remove deep-seated hurts, habits and addictions. This is very difficult because reaching the core of consciousness requires peeling off the layers of the mind, which are numerous and complex.

Once our deeper consciousness is disturbed, which is a trauma to the heart, it is very difficult to regain psychological equilibrium. We must nurture our consciousness with higher impulses, not expose it to negative influences from the external world. Our core consciousness is the mind of the child that takes in everything and must be protected.

Composition

Conditioned consciousness (Chitta) is primarily Sattvic in nature but contains all three gunas in their seed forms. The essence of the three gunas within us determines the nature of our deeper consciousness. It is composed of the gunas that we most hold to in our hearts. Our relationships at a heart level most affect our consciousness and transmit their gunas to us.

Consciousness becomes purely sattvic and fully developed as the result of spiritual practice. Otherwise its function is inhibited and distorted. Rajas and Tamas (aggression and ignorance) in consciousness cause pain and delusion and are the source of all problems in life. These are the main psychological impurities or toxins that we must eliminate. Our deeper consciousness is the level at which these mental toxins reside and the seat from which they have to be removed.

Tamas in the Chitta becomes the unconscious, which

dominates us during sleep, dullness and depression. It is
the basis of the habits and tendencies that we know are
wrong but are unable to change with our surface mind.
Rajas in the Chitta underlies our usual waking consciousness, characterized by action and expression. It keeps our
consciousness ever moving, disturbed and distracted,
caught up in its own imaginings. Sattva in the Chitta provides the basis for our higher conscious and superconscious
functioning.

Chitta constitutes the causal body, the reincarnating
vehicle of the individual soul that persists through the
entire cycle of rebirth. It contains the karmic residues set
in motion in various lives, only a few of which come to the
surface and manifest in any particular incarnation. As the
causal or creative venture, consciousness contains the
potential for all developments of body and mind. It is the
source of the five sensory potentials and the five gross elements, which create and sustain the subtle and gross bodies. Chitta is desire predominant[17] and is the basis of the
core desires that keep us in the cycle of rebirth.

The field of consciousness (Chitta) makes up the Anandamaya kosha or bliss sheath in which we carry our deepest joys and sorrows. In its unawakened (Tamasic) condition the Anandamaya kosha is the repository of our
clinging to embodied existence. In its awakened (Sattvic)
state it reflects the bliss inherent in our Self that is one
with God.

Relative to the five elements, Chitta most corresponds
to air and ether. Its substance is like ether, its motion like
air. Like air, it is ever changing and adjusting itself both
inwardly and outwardly, ever expansive and creative. Consciousness, like air, is ever contacting things and making
sound. Consciousness is nothing but the inmost core of

sound vibrating within us. Chitta transcends the senses but has a special connection with the sense of hearing, particularly non-verbalized sound and music. Sound influences and heals the Chitta, a point we will examine under Mantra Therapy.

Though Chitta is much more subtle than the biological humors, Chitta generally relates to Vata, the most primary of these. Vata people live with an exposed consciousness or vulnerable heart. Their consciousness is open and they are less grounded in their bodies and senses. For this reason, Vata-types are more easily hurt than others and should be treated with care. Keeping Vata in balance protects and aids in the proper unfoldment of our deeper consciousness. Similarly, Chitta corresponds to Prana among the three vital essences.

Energy/Will

Chitta governs the original Prana, the immortal life-force of the soul through which we are animate or alive on all levels. Just as it relates to the Gunas in general, so does it relate to the Pranas, and also corresponds to Prana among the three vital essences (Prana, Tejas and Ojas). This master Prana gives life to the mind and the body and upholds all autonomic functions. Nothing is dearer to us than life itself, which takes us to the bliss inherent within us.

Consciousness holds the original life-force that is the reflection of the eternal and immortal life of the Supreme Self. Because of its deep connection with the life-force, the practice of Pranayama can help us enter into and purify the Chitta. What alternative medicine calls the "intelligence of the body" is the hidden aspect of Chitta working in the body. When we give up ego control, it can function without obstruction to heal and rejuvenate us physically and mentally.

Consciousness holds the deepest level of will, which is the will to live, the desire to exist forever. Our deeper consciousness holds our most primal and ultimate motivations, our heart's desires and wishes, what we really want in life. Consciousness is will in the general and potential sense — pure will without a defined goal, the will to experience that is the basis of all other intentions. From it arises all the desires that keep us bound to the world and to the body. Only if we gain freedom from these core desires can we perceive the truth.

Consciousness and Individual Nature

The fabric of our consciousness consists of deep-seated thought tendencies called Samskaras in Sanskrit. These are deeper than what we ordinarily regard as thoughts. They are the residues that we retain from our mental operations, like the ruts a turning wheel makes in a road. These residues support the behavioral patterns that motivate us from within.

What we call the nature or being of the individual is the consciousness of the person. Our individual consciousness is the field of the tendencies that we have made our own, the ground of our repeated actions that have become automatic or second nature. Our conditioning in life creates the state or condition of our consciousness. It is our deepest level of programming. Our existence is our consciousness which determines how we relate to life. The state of the Chitta or core consciousness is the mental natur (Manasika Prakrit) of the person and determines our unique character and mentality.

The nature of a person cannot be changed without

changing the deeper consciousness, which means to change the heart. Unless an influence gets to the level of the heart, it cannot have any deep or lasting effect. This is why mere words or thoughts have such little value. They do not go beyond the surface mind in their effects. Yet to get to the core of the heart requires uncovering all our sorrows and regrets, which most of us are unwilling to face.

Functions

All the functions of the mind are functions of the Chitta, which constitutes the entire mental field. However, Chitta has three general functions, which are three primary ways to access this deeper consciousness. To reach these we must withdraw from the outer mind and senses which keep our awareness on the surface of our being. These three are: 1) memory; 2) sleep; and 3) samadhi.

Memory

Consciousness is the ground of memory and consists primarily of memories. It includes not only the ordinary memory of information but what we really remember in our hearts, those things that most deeply affect us for good or ill. It holds our seed memories from life to life. Our deeper consciousness governs memory on an organic level, including the memory that exists in our cells, through which the body functions. Our consciousness even has the capacity to remember God and to remember that we are God because, as consciousness, in its core is the soul which reflects God. Our consciousness can remember the entire universe, which after all is a formation of consciousness.

Memory can give us either bondage or liberation. True memory is self-remembrance, remembering our Divine nature in consciousness. False memory is memory of personal joys and sorrows, the history of the ego. The best way to develop memory is to memorize truth principles and higher cosmic laws.[18]

Sleep

In sleep, the outer world shuts off and we return to the inner world of consciousness. Impressions arise as dreams through the activity of the subtle mind. Generally, the predominant impressions of daily activity get illumined, but sometimes deeper samskaras arise. Consciousness in its right function gives peaceful deep sleep. Disturbed by Rajas and Tamas, it creates bad dreams and restless sleep.

In sleep, our mind gets renewed by immersion in its source, our core consciousness which contains the primal Prana or life-force. Consciousness and Prana sustain the involuntary functions of the body, while the mind and senses rest.

Death is a prolonged sleep. Like sleep, it is an immersion in our inner consciousness in which we lose contact with the outer world of the senses. In the sleep of death, consciousness holds the causal Prana and the karmas from which a new body will be created. In death, we dwell in consciousness only and renew ourselves for another birth.

In the after-death state, the impressions of our life-experience arise from our inner consciousness, much like dreams. This creates various subtle or astral worlds, like the heavens and hells, which the subtle mind visualizes. These are good or bad according to our karma and life-experience.

Samadhi

Samadhi is a state of absorption in which our consciousness becomes entirely concentrated in a single object or experience and we forget all other things. Yogic practice aims at developing absorption in Cosmic Consciousness and in our true Self. Through it, consciousness is put to rest in the higher sense, providing lasting peace and liberation. The higher development of the consciousness occurs only through Samadhi. Awareness of the deeper levels of consciousness in Samadhi neutralizes our karmas and releases us from the cycle of birth and death.

However, Samadhi includes not only spiritual states but any peak experience. Any experience in which we become so immersed that we forget ourselves is a kind of Samadhi. There are inferior Samadhis, or absorptions of the disturbed or darkened consciousness in which Rajas and Tamas prevail. When the mind becomes concentrated in anything, including negative emotions like fear or anger, we move to some degree into our deeper consciousness. These negative absorptions, however, increase our bondage to the external world and should be avoided. They increase Rajas and Tamas, while spiritual absorptions increase Sattva.[19]

Additional Functions

From these primary functions, different secondary functions evolve.

Intuition

Consciousness in its higher function becomes intuition, which is the capacity to know things directly. Through intuition, we feel within ourselves what we may have never contacted through our senses. True intuition is a kind of Samadhi. As the direct feeling of consciousness, it can be more vivid than sensory knowledge. We should not confuse it with imagination or psychic perception, however, which are functions of the outer mind and subtle senses.

Instinct

In its lower function, consciousness becomes instinct, which sustains our organic functions and protects them from interference from the ego. Instinct is a secret or hidden form of higher knowledge, or intuition inverted. Consciousness governs all instinctual responses. On its level deep, instinctual patterns abide, like survival or reproduction, which are therefore very hard to change. Changing our core consciousness requires making the unconscious, automatic or instinctual part of the mind conscious and aware.

Love

The basic urge of consciousness is to unite. It consists of our efforts and energies to unite either outwardly with the world or inwardly with our true nature. To "be" is to be related through consciousness. Through consciousness, we relate to the world and the world is related to us, not merely superficially but at a heart level. Through love's capacity of sympathy and rapport, consciousness creates devotion and compassion, the guiding powers of the spiritual life.

Consciousness is the basis of love, which is the essential attitude and energy of the heart. In fact, consciousness is love. On individual consciousness the Divine Consciousness projects its power of eternal and unbounded love. Love derives from consciousness, which is its home. Consciousness is the love at the core of our being. In its internal fount of love, we find complete and perfect happiness, which arises through being able to be one with the object of our love.

Faith

Our deeper consciousness is the basis of real faith which, like intuition, is a direct inner sense of Reality that lies beyond all appearances. This true faith of the heart possesses an inherent knowledge of the Eternal and the Infinite, and is quite apart from any dogma. When we give our faith over to a particular dogma — restricting truth to a person, book, or institution — the ability of consciousness to reflect the truth becomes distorted. Whatever we have faith in enters into the deeper levels of consciousness (the heart).

Our beliefs are our most deep-seated thoughts and unquestioned preconceptions. They are our deepest tendencies and samskaras. Our core beliefs adhere in our core consciousness, coloring every mental activity. To really change our consciousness requires giving up these unquestioned beliefs by changing how we feel in our hearts.

Proper Development

The proper development of consciousness requires its deconditioning. For this, we must release the deep-seated desires, habits and tendencies stored within it. This is only possible through Samadhi or absorption in truth. Yet, to be able to decondition consciousness, first requires that we put our outer lives into the proper order. Consciousness must be brought to a purely sattvic state of peace and openness.

All factors that purify and calm the mind aid in this development, including right diet, proper impressions, right action and right relationship. Ayurvedic psychology aims at the proper development of consciousness so that we can go beyond the problems of the mind, which are all caused by unconsciousness or lack of awareness. Then we

can complete our journey from conditioned consciousness
to pure awareness, in which nothing external can any
longer cause us sorrow.

7. Intelligence:
The Power of Perception

Intelligence is the flame of truth that illumines our lives; how we cultivate it determines the light by which we live and grow, or the darkness by which we become narrow and decay. We all wish to become more aware and understanding, but what is true intelligence and how can we develop it? Not only Ayurveda but all true psychology revolves around this as its central point.

If we have not developed our intelligence properly, we misuse the body and senses. Dietary and lifestyle indiscretions follow, which weaken our vitality and hasten the aging process. Emotional disturbances and mental afflictions increase. On the other hand, if we use our intelligence properly, we respect our bodies and the world around us and use things wisely and appropriately. We develop a way of life that allows us to live better and longer, not merely for our own sake but for the good of others. We strive to control our thoughts and emotions. Hence we must strive to develop our intelligence, or like a dim light it will lead us into error.[20]

The Sanskrit term for intelligence is Buddhi, deriving from the root "bud," which means "to perceive" or "to become awake." Buddhi is the aspect of consciousness that is filled with light and reveals the truth. When one's Buddhi becomes fully developed, one becomes a Buddha or enlightened one.[21] The main action of intelligence is to discern the true and real from the false and unreal. It enables us to discriminate the nature of things from mere appearances or speculations. Through it we develop our core perceptions of self and world: who we are, why we exist, and what the world is.

Intelligence: Abstract and Concrete

Intelligence is the objective part of the mind capable of detached observation. Its concrete side allows us to grasp external objects, while its abstract side enables us to comprehend ideas. Its concrete side tells us the particular object that we see is a man, a horse, a house, or whatever it may be. Through its abstract side, we recognize the qualities and values an object may represent, its truth or worth.

The concrete side of intelligence produces science, along with all forms of sensory-based knowledge and all systems of measurement. Its abstract side creates philosophy, through which we can perceive universals and know the ideal form of things. Through its abstract side, intelligence can conceive of the Divine or infinite and becomes the basis of spirituality.

Intelligence and Intellect

Intelligence has a dual capacity, according to whether we direct it outwardly or inwardly. The nature of its orientation is the key to evolution in humanity. Intelligence functioning outwardly through the senses becomes "intellect," the concrete or informational side of intelligence. Functioning inwardly through our deeper consciousness, it becomes what could be better called "true intelligence." The distinction between intellect and true intelligence is crucial for understanding the condition of the world today and essential for establishing any real depth psychology.

Intellect refers to an intelligence that uses reason, based upon the senses, to determine truth. It extends the range of the senses through various instruments, like telescopes and microscopes, and increases its calculating capacity through various machines, like computers. It invents different systems of ideas, temporal and spatial measurements, to understand the world.

Intellect constructs the idea of an external world as reality, noting the names and forms of things in the world and placing them into various categories and hierarchies. The notion of an outer world of enjoyment as our place of fulfillment derives from it. From it comes a materialistic view of life and a mechanistic view of the universe. Intellect directs us to outer goals in life: enjoyment, wealth, power or mundane knowledge. It creates a bodily idea of existence, in which we become trapped in time and space, sorrow and death. Intellect emphasizes outer distinctions, roles, and identities. Through it we get caught in surface information, status and possessions. Intellect functions under the control of ego and emotion rather than guiding them. It can inhibit our spiritual evolution, making us prefer solid worldly realities over inner experiences.

True intelligence is a power of inner or direct perception quite different from the secondhand or mediated knowledge of the intellect. It reveals to us the nature of things, transcending their sensory appearances, the content behind the often misleading package. True intelligence takes the eternal to be the real, and perceives transient names and forms as unreal. Through it we go beyond all beliefs, preconceptions, and concepts and learn to see things as they are.

True intelligence is keenly aware of the impermanence

of all external reality and does not attach us to any fixed names and forms. Through it we learn to perceive the consciousness behind the shifting movements of matter and energy in the external world. We free ourselves from outer belief structures, authorities and institutions, transcending time and space into the reality of our True Nature.

The intellect possesses only an indirect knowledge or mediated knowledge of names, numbers and appearances. For this reason, the intellect cannot solve our human problems or bring peace to the psyche. It is not enough to know what our problems are conceptually. We must understand their origin in our own hearts and souls. Without an awakening of true intelligence, our society must remain emotionally unstable and spiritually naive. Western psychology, with some exceptions, shares the limitations of an intellectual view of life that the West has generally glorified in its philosophy and science. Ayurveda, based on Yogic philosophy, regards the intellect as a lower or inferior intelligence. It helps us cultivate our deeper intelligence, which takes us beyond the senses to the truth within our hearts.

Conscience

Each of us possesses an inherent ethical sense, which we call "conscience" — a feeling that certain things are right and others are wrong. Our conscience causes us not to wish harm to any creature and to feel the pain of others as our own. Conscience is a major part of intelligence, which establishes how we value and treat other people. The more intelligent we are, the stronger a conscience we have and the less we seek to interfere with others or impose our will upon them.

Directly outwardly, intelligence creates morality, which

may be little more than the arbitrary customs of a particular society. Directed inwardly, intelligence creates universal ethics like non-violence, which transcend all cultural prejudices. Through our inner intelligence, we act ethically and humanely, not for material or social gain, or even for heavenly reward, but for the good of all.

Organized religion, with its dogmas and institutions, is another product of the outward-oriented intelligence. It results in the clash of beliefs and their exclusive claims. It ties us to a particular church, book or savior as truth. On the other hand, directed inwardly, true intelligence creates spirituality or the quest for eternal truth beyond name and form. It leads to the truth of our own inner Being, our higher Self in which the insistence upon a belief, savior or institution appears naive.

Intelligence and Awareness

True intelligence is the aspect of consciousness that is awake, cognizant, and developed, while consciousness (Chitta) itself is the mental field as a whole, particularly its undeveloped core. Consciousness, as it evolves, turns into intelligence that articulates and clarifies it. Consciousness, when directed toward a particular principle, value, or higher good, becomes intelligence. In its highest function, intelligence becomes spiritual discrimination,[22] through which we discern the inner reality from outer forms, which releases our consciousness from its negative conditioning.

Consciousness contains everything in the mental field in a potential or seed form. Intelligence allows us to become aware of the contents of consciousness, which otherwise lie hidden and unperceived. The cultivation of awareness, which is meditation, is necessary to develop true intelligence. However, the mind's intelligence (Buddhi) is always an awareness of something and remains conditioned by its object. We must eventually step beyond it to discover our true Self (Atman) beyond the mind. The Self is the origin of intelligence. The reflection of its unconditioned intelligence endows the mental field with a conditioned intelligence. Our conditioned intelligence is an instrument for the unconditioned intelligence of the Self. From conditioned consciousness and intelligence (Chitta and Buddhi), we must move to unconditioned conscious and intelligence (Chit and Jnana).

Cosmic Intelligence

Intelligence has a cosmic as well as individual reality.[23] Cosmic Intelligence is the evolved or sattvic portion of Cosmic Consciousness. It is the mind of God at the summit of creation, through which God functions as the Creator-Preserver-Destroyer of the universe.[24] Cosmic Intelligence is the field of God's action, the manifestation of His laws. It is the Divine Word, the Logos, through which the universe is created. From it comes the first or ideal creation, of which this material world is an imperfect reflection.

Cosmic Intelligence is responsible for the structure and order of the cosmos, while Cosmic Consciousness governs the world process and being. A portion of Cosmic Intelligence descends into matter and becomes the Divine flame that constructs the worlds.[25] Our individual intelligence is our particular portion of Cosmic Intelligence or the Divine Word. This Divine flame is ever awake at the deepest level of our consciousness as our inner guide.[26] It directs our evolutionary process from matter to spirit, from the unconscious to the superconscious, from ignorance to enlightenment. Cosmic Intelligence is the inner guru who works to awaken our internal wisdom.

Cosmic Intelligence contains all cosmic laws (Dharmas), from those that govern the physical world to the ethical principles that govern our karma. It is the field of natural law, in which all the laws of life are held. Our individual intelligence naturally strives to learn the laws of Cosmic Intelligence, through which the entire universe can be comprehended. Cosmic Intelligence establishes what is dharmic, or in harmony with cosmic law, as opposed to what is adharmic, or contrary to it. Individual intelligence grows through aligning itself with Cosmic Intelligence that is its source. This happens not by mere study of books, but by studying nature and, above all, by observing oneself.

Composition

True intelligence develops from sattvic or finer matters of consciousness (Chitta). However, directed outwardly, intelligence becomes contaminated with rajas, or emotional impurities, which cloud its perception,[27] and by tamas, which causes wrong judgment.

The seat of true intelligence, like that of consciousness, resides in the heart. However, the seat of intellect, or outer intelligence, is the brain, which is connected with the senses. Intelligence mediates between the outer mind that works through the brain and the inner mind located in the heart.[28] To merge intelligence into the heart is the way to transcend the outer world and return to the inner Self. This is the basis of all true meditation.

The field of intelligence makes up the sheath of intelligence or wisdom, Vijnanamaya Kosha. This sheath mediates between the causal (karmic) body and the astral or subtle body of impressions. Without the proper development of the intelligence sheath, the potentials of the deeper bliss sheath (Anandamaya Kosha) cannot develop. It serves as the door that links the outer world of the mind-body complex with the senses and the inner world of consciousness, which transcends the senses. Intelligence is knowledge predominant[29] and allows us to understand things.

Intelligence adds the power of fire to the basic ether and air elements of consciousness (Chitta). Like fire, it is penetrating, luminous and transformative in action. Intelligence corresponds to Pitta, or fire, among the biological humors. Pitta people are usually rational, discriminating, good speakers, and usually have more perceptive minds than others, for good or ill. Similarly, intelligence relates to Tejas, the vital fire essence which provides courage, fearlessness and determination. Without Tejas, we lack the independence and clarity necessary to develop our intelligence properly.

Energy/Awakened Prana

By its sattvic nature, intelligence transcends outward vital and sensory activity and works as the conscious guide of all the Pranas. It creates sattvic Prana or conscious use of our life-energy. Intelligence has the power to control the mind, senses and vital force, according to its experiential knowledge. For example, once we have really learned that walking across the street without looking puts us in danger of being run over, we will not fail to look when we cross the street, even if we are in a hurry. The problem is that if our intelligence is not developed properly, it is dominated by the mind, senses and vital force and we do things on impulse that later we must regret. This inability of intelligence to control our impulses is one of the main causes of disease.[30]

True intelligence relates to what we have learned not merely theoretically but in our own life-experience and behavior. It is the wisdom of life. On the other hand, what we know merely conceptually has no real vitality. It reflects life on the outside, imitating the ideas and opinions of others, and cannot change us fundamentally. The energy of intelligence is the power that we place in knowledge — the Prana we direct toward discovering the truth. The Prana of intelligence is ever awake and attuned to the eternal, developing the aspirations of our soul.

In yogic practice, Prana begins to awaken. We experience expanded energy through the breath, or feel various currents of energy moving through the body, awakening our subtle faculties. We gain more energy, enthusiasm and creativity. This Prana has an intelligence that can teach and guide us. Prana has become the teacher of many yogis and has taught them asana, mantra and meditation. Surrendering to that awakened Prana becomes their discipline. Yet we must be careful not to surrender to an inferior Prana, or inferior vital urge, which is what we do when we are pursuing outer enjoyment, but to discover the Prana of intelligence (Buddhi-Prana).

The awakened Prana and the awakened intelligence (Buddhi) are related. As Buddhi awakens, so does Prana. As our Prana awakens, so does Buddhi. The awakened life and awakened intelligence move together. Intelligence purifies and clarifies our life. On the other hand, without vitality our intelligence remains superficial and theoretical. The wisdom of life is this unity of Buddhi and Prana.

Will — The Doer

Intelligence is the agent or doer that decides what we must do. Only when we really know are we capable of making a decision and doing something. Intelligence is the executive part of consciousness, the commander who is responsible for determining our line of action. The mind and body are its instruments. Intelligence establishes lasting goals and provides the knowledge to achieve them; the mind executes its orders through the body and senses.

Intelligence is will in the higher sense — the will to truth, the will to realize our ideals or achieve our goals.[31] It is the basis of spiritual aspiration, the desire to know God. Our intelligence determines what we should and should not do, providing the ethical standard for our behavior. As intelligence develops, we move away from lower actions and embrace those that are higher. Intelligence holds the striving of our soul toward enlightenment.

True intelligence leads us to selfless service, in which we act for the good of all and renounce the fruits of our deeds. Through it we are dedicated to excellence and strive to do the best, whatever the consequences. Intelligence acts with clarity and decisiveness to achieve a higher aim and ceases from action once it achieves its purpose. In this regard it is the clear action that leads to inaction or peace. From it come proficiency and mastery in all fields of life, including spiritual accomplishments and occult powers. Through it we can master our destiny and transcend the world.

At the time of death, the senses merge into the mind and the mind, in turn, merges into intelligence, which, as our inner flame, takes us to whatever subtle world our karma merits. According to the values and goals of the intelligence, the soul moves on to various after-death states, and then returns for another physical birth. As is our intelligence, so is our will, so is our karma and the evolution of our soul. Our higher intelligence alone can endure consciously from life to life. Whatever power-of-truth intelligence we develop can never leave us. Developing it should be the main goal of all that we do. For this reason, the soul and intelligence are closely related. True intelligence is the mind of soul, its awakened perception.

Functions

The main function of intelligence is determination of truth, which occurs in three ways: 1) perception; 2) reason; and 3) testimony.

Perception

Direct perception is the main way that we determine the nature of objects. It allows us to identify the enduring realities behind various shifting sensory impressions. The capacity of the sense organs to perceive comes from the working of intelligence. Right functioning of the senses depends upon their alignment with intelligence, which frees them from emotional distortion and brings into them the clarity of awareness.

Intelligence allows us to differentiate what objects are from what we would like them to be, the Real from the imaginary. Through it we can perceive sensations, emotions, thoughts, and the ego itself, just as we can perceive objects in the external world. Functioning wrongly, however, intelligence results in distorted or erroneous perception. We mistake one thing for another, like confusing a rope in the dark for a snake. This creates all the errors, misconceptions and wrong judgments that trouble us.

Reason

Intelligence governs all reasoning methods, inductive and deductive. It allows us to compare our impressions and arrive at a greater truth, like deducing fire from the presence of smoke. From it come the principles, ideals and systems of measurement that shape our perceptions and guide our actions. In its wrong function, intelligence causes false reasoning or rationalization, through which we try to justify what is false or illusory. This egoistic intelligence is perhaps the greatest danger for human beings, because it turns the instrument of truth into one of self-justification that shuts off any real learning process.

Testimony

Intelligence governs our ability to listen, to heed the advice of others. It gives the ability to learn, which comes from right listening. A good intelligence makes a good student, disciple or patient. Wrongly functioning, intelligence makes us deaf to advice or words of good counsel. True intelligence is the guru, adviser, and teacher. It is the speaker, the one who speaks not merely casually or gives his impressions, but who declares what he knows to be the truth. From Cosmic Intelligence comes the scripture or Word of Truth that sets forth the truth and how to realize it. All spiritual teachings come from the higher levels of intelligence.

Sound has the ability to convey knowledge of the invisible and transcendent. On the ordinary level, it can convey knowledge of other times and places. On a higher level, it reminds us of the knowledge inherent in our soul. While higher realities like God or the Self are not known to the outer mind, their knowledge is inherent in our hearts and can be awakened by the right words aligned with the love and wisdom of the speaker. In this regard, sound and speech are more important means of knowledge than are sensory perception and reason, but for this to occur our minds and hearts must be open to the inner truth.

Intelligence relates to the organ of speech among the vocal organs, and the organ of hearing among the sense organs. These are the most rational and spiritual of the organs, the most free from the limitations of form, through which we can contact our inner intelligence. Sound itself is a means of direct and internal knowledge, while other sensory knowledge remains limited to the outer.

ADDITIONAL FUNCTIONS

Wakefulness

Intelligence governs the waking state in which clear perception occurs. It predominates in human beings who represent the waking state of consciousness, and distinguishes the human from the animal and vegetable kingdoms. Intelligence is responsible for wakefulness as a whole. Our degree of spiritual wakefulness is the measure of how we have developed our intelligence.

Intelligence gives directed awareness, through which we can concentrate fully on a particular object. Consciousness (Chitta), on the other hand, gives open or choiceless awareness, through which the whole can be grasped. While memory abides in consciousness, clarity of memory belongs to intelligence. Intelligence gives us objective recall of events. The ability to remember what we know, without which knowledge is of little value, is the ability of intelligence to access consciousness. Without such memory, our intelligence cannot develop properly. When the time comes to use our knowledge without such memory, we will not have access to it. For this reason cultivation of memory is a key to the development of intelligence.

Samadhi

Samadhi is the fourth and highest means of knowledge, and is the ultimate form of direct perception. It occurs when intelligence uses our deeper consciousness as its instrument of perception. This only happens when we transcend the intellect into true intelligence.[32] It requires that the senses are silent and we can look within without distraction. Then, by the light of our own consciousness, we can discover all the secrets of life.

Spiritual practice consists of converting the raw material of consciousness into the refined energy of intelligence. Awareness in consciousness is general and rudimentary, while in intelligence it is fully developed and articulate. Intelligence illumines our deeper consciousness, which in turn gives it space and depth. Intelligence takes us from the unconscious to the superconscious, from sleep to Samadhi. Meditation is the highest function of intelligence. True intelligence creates Samadhi and immerses us in our deeper consciousness in an attentive way.[33]

Samadhis, which involve concentration, one-pointedness of mind and directed mental activity, belong to intelligence. Higher Samadhis, in which there is no thought or action, and the mind is not one-pointed but calmed, are of the deeper consciousness. In these, intelligence ceases to have any separate function and intelligence and consciousness become one. This takes us into the unconditioned in which all thoughts disappear.

Proper Development

To develop true intelligence requires placing the intellect in the service of awareness. This occurs when we recognize the difference between the higher and the lower knowledge, which is the distinction between self-knowledge and knowledge of externals. Through the lower, we understand the outer world and how it functions, but this knowledge remains bound to the realm of form and change. Through the higher knowledge, we know ourselves. Our true nature is eternal consciousness that cannot be determined by the names and forms of outer knowing. Our immortal Self is the knower. It cannot be an object of the mind but is the origin of the mind. We can only know it by being it.

There is nothing wrong with the intellect as long as we keep it in its place. We all need a clear intellect to deal with the practical realities of everyday existence, like driving a car. But if the outer function of intellect is not balanced by the inner function of intelligence, it leads to distortion and can become destructive. Ayurvedic psychological methods bring about the proper development of intelligence so that we can perceive our problems and their causes, and change them in a lasting manner. The language and tools of Ayurveda are not merely man-made, but reflect Cosmic Intelligence and help us attune our life and behavior to it.

8. The Outer Mind:
The Field of the Senses

Our lives revolve around the vast array of sensory impressions that are ever coming to us from the external world. At almost every moment of the day we are engaged in selecting, filtering and organizing this data and seeing what it means for our welfare and happiness. We are seldom aware of our minds because we are always using them to deal with the external world and its demands. Like a car we are always driving, we do not have the time to stop and see if it is working properly, unless it breaks down. It is mainly in the outer, sensory part of the mind that we live, unless we learn to look within.

Our ordinary awareness remains immersed in the sea of impressions that constantly streams in through the senses. Most of what we call the mind is this surface part of consciousness through which we handle impressions. This outer mind is called Manas in Sanskrit,[34] which means the "instrument of thinking." Manas is the most complex aspect of consciousness, consisting of the senses, emotions, and outer thinking capacity. Such diversity is necessary for dealing with the manifold influences of the external world.

We will refer to Manas as the "outer" or "sense mind," or as simply "mind" itself, as opposed to "intelligence" (Buddhi) and "inner mind" or "consciousness" (Chitta). However, we should not forget their Sanskrit meanings.

Including emotion, mind (Manas) is not simply mental or conceptual.

The Five Senses and Motor Organs

We possess five senses and five motor organs through which we take in the energies of the five elements and act upon them in the outer world.

SENSE AND MOTOR ORGANS

Element	Humor	Sense Quality	Sense Organ	Motor Organ
Ether	Vata	Sound	Ears	Vocal Organ
Air	Vata	Touch	Skin	Hands
Fire	Pitta	Sight	Eyes	Feet
Water	Kapha	Taste	Tongue	Reproductive Organs
Earth	Kapha	Smell	Nose	Organs of Elimination

The mind coordinates the five senses and their data. It functions as the screen on which sensory data is gathered and scrutinized. Through the mind, for example, what the eye sees is correlated with what the ear hears. Otherwise, the data coming in from the different senses would remain separate and disorganized.

The mind itself is the sixth sense organ because through it we take in ideas and emotions — mental impressions. When we read a book, for example, the mind is also functioning as a sense organ, taking in emotional and mental information. All our sensory inputs involve some mental and emotional component. Similarly, the mind is the sixth motor organ and rules over the other five. As an organ of action, it is our main means of expression in the outer world. Only what we have first formulated as a mental intention can we express through our motor organs. For example, we must first think of what to say before we actually speak. As an organ of action, the mind serves to express ideas and emotions — mental conditions.

As a sense and a motor organ, the mind can coordinate the two types of organs, connecting sensory data with motor actions. For example, if we see food on the table, the mind connects that sensory data with the hands to allow us to pick up the food and eat it. The mind is the central circuit board for both sensory and motor organs. It is like our mental computer, while the senses are its software.

Though the mind relates to both sense and motor organs, it connects more with the motor organs because its main concern is action in the outer world. The mind is ever driving us to do things. It is ever thinking, planning, reacting emotionally or otherwise seeking to engage us externally. Through it we are conscious of ourselves as beings in the world.

The Pranas

Both motor and sense organs are closely aligned to Prana and its functions. The motor organs exist to fulfill various vital urges, from eating to self-expression. The sense organs exist to provide knowledge and experience of the external world. The mind manages the Pranas, operating through the sense and motor organs. The mind is influenced by the Pranas and can easily be disturbed by them. Whatever affects our vital nature, like hunger, fear or insult, quickly affects the mind.

The senses possess their own instincts and energies that can dominate the mind. The eye has the urge to see, the tongue the urge to taste, the hands the urge to grasp, and so on. These urges influence the mind to pursue their aims. The eyes can tell the mind what to see, for example, as when the image of a beautiful woman draws the mind of a man outward automatically. This happens to all of us with one sense organ or another. We are always struggling to control our senses, which otherwise would fragment our awareness.

Animals are dominated by their sensory impulses. For example, a dog barks automatically when another dog comes into its sensory field. The sense mind predominates in children, who have not yet learned to master their sensory capacities. The outer mind is conditioned through the sense organs and Pranas. In itself it is largely a reaction mechanism, not a self-aware consciousness which only comes through intelligence.

Thought and Emotion: The Two Sides of the Mind

The outer mind does not merely coordinate sensory data, but interprets it. Sensory data, being potentially endless, must be filtered and selected according to what is relevant for the mind. We determine this by where we place our attention. For example, if we are driving a car, we must give our attention to the road and not let it wander or we might get into an accident.

Interpretation of sensory data is twofold — both objective and subjective. Objectively we organize sensory data, gathering in the proper impressions to determine their meaning. To identify an object, like a house, for example, we must take in enough objective impressions to ascertain its nature. This creates the factual part of the mind. The outer mind governs factual information and data of all types, much like a computer. This it transfers on to the Buddhi for judgment.

Subjectively, we must relate sensory data to our own personal condition. For example, when we are crossing a street and see that a car may hit us, we react quickly to protect ourselves, getting scared and moving aside. This creates the emotional part of the mind. Emotion allows us to respond to sensory data in an immediate and personal manner. Emotion is our personal reaction to sensory data, giving us fear of what causes pain and desire for what brings pleasure.

The outer mind includes thought of an informational nature and emotion based on sensation and functions between the two. We need some degree of objectivity to organize sensory data, but some degree of subjectivity to relate it to ourselves. Of the mind's two functions, emotion, which is subjective, has the greatest capacity for causing pain. Emotion can distort the informational capacity of the mind and create misperception. The emotional side of the mind connects more with the Pranas and the motor organs, which serve mainly to fulfill various Pranic activities. The mental side connects more with the sensory organs and intelligence.

Emotion

Emotions are characterized by a sensory component — the sights, sounds or other sensations that convey them. Sensation gives rise to emotion. If we contact something pleasurable, it makes us happy. If we contact something painful, we feel sad. This emotional vulnerability is built into the mind.

Temporary emotional reactions come through the outer

mind. Enduring emotional states, however, belong to our deeper consciousness (Chitta). Repeated emotions move from reactions of the outer mind into conditions of the inner consciousness. For example, when we first meet an attractive partner, our emotion is aroused. After we've been in a long-term relationship, the person becomes part of our deeper consciousness, and we take on aspects of his or her personality.

Specific emotions, tied to particular objects, belong to the outer mind, but the essence of emotion belongs to our deeper consciousness. There the moods or flavors (rasas) of emotions dwell — like love, anger, fear, and joy — beyond any association with particular sensations.[35] For this reason, both those who hold that emotions are more superficial than thought and those who hold they are deeper are both correct. It depends upon the type of emotion. I prefer to call these deeper emotions of our core consciousness "feelings" and use the term emotion or emotional reactions for the emotions of the outer mind.

Outer Mind and Intelligence

The outer mind allows us to register information. Intelligence allows us to process information. The mind (Manas) is the instrument of thinking in which we entertain doubts, while intelligence (Buddhi) is the instrument of perception through which we resolve doubts and make decisions. The outer mind includes all forms of speculation and imagination. As long as we are on the outer level of the mind, we must remain in doubt and susceptible to emotional reactions. People who are good at gathering information but poor at making decisions suffer from too much activity of the mind. The mind working apart from intelligence causes us to think aimlessly, without purpose, as in daydreaming, idle speculation or idle calculation. It causes us to go over ideas, generally useless, without coming to any conclusion, which requires the action of intelligence.

The outer mind itself has no values, principles or goals, which derive from intelligence. Its concern is expansion and exploration of the external world, seeking pleasure and avoiding pain. Its purpose is to afford us experience in the realm of the senses, not to establish lasting values. As long as we operate on its level, we are purely sensate creatures. We are victims of the emotions aroused by our senses — the attraction to pleasurable sensations and the aversion to painful ones.

Our modern information-sensation culture is dominated by the outer mind and lacking in intelligence. We are more concerned with gathering information through the mind than with digesting it, which requires intelligence. We have developed many ways to expand the field of sensory data, but not the wisdom to use it properly.

Though the sense organs function through the mind, which coordinates their activity, sensory perception, like all forms of perception, occurs through intelligence (Buddhi). The mind holds the images of objects but intelligence definitively ascertains what they are. Only when intelligence guides the senses can we use them objectively. For this reason, the sense organs are sometimes included in the sphere of intelligence.

Intelligence is the inner or subjective part of the mind through which we make choices and decisions. The outer mind is the screen on which we perceive the external world and execute these choices and decisions. Intelligence therefore draws us within, while the mind draws us externally. The purpose of the outer mind is enjoyment (bhoga), which is externally directed. Spiritual development (yoga), whose movement is within, arises only through the power of intelligence. While the mind leads us to worldly involvement, intelligence leads us to spiritual development. However, in the evolved state, the mind allows us to respond creatively to external influences. It becomes the basis of right action, without which we could not organize our outer lives according to any higher principles.

Mind, Intelligence and Consciousness

Consciousness (Chitta) feels internally and has its own sense of knowing. The mind (Manas) senses things outwardly, requiring an external impression for it to function. Intelligence (Buddhi) perceives and recognizes both inwardly and outwardly. For example, through the mind one may sense a person is unhappy, an impression that comes through putting together the information of the senses. Through intelligence, one will perceive it as an objective fact, by reasoning based upon what one sees. Through one's deeper consciousness, one will actually feel the unhappiness of the other person.

The outer mind, relying upon the senses, gives a sense of something, which usually remains tinged with doubt. Intelligence perceives an object, depending upon some rational process, in which there is no longer any doubt. Consciousness feels the object as one's own.

Intelligence (Buddhi) and consciousness (Chitta) only function in our ordinary awareness through the outer mind and senses (Manas), in which we are usually engaged. Such intelligence or intellect only serves to discriminate the names and forms recognized by the outer mind. Such consciousness only serves to heighten the sensations received through the outer mind.

Cosmic Mind

Collective and cosmic counterparts of the mind exist as well. Its collective side is the sensory activity of other creatures on Earth. The sensory influences of creatures create the psychic atmosphere in which we function. Sensory impressions leave a residue or afterglow. The Earth's atmosphere is filled with the residual sensory impressions of creatures. The mass media is filling the psychic atmosphere with unwholesome impressions in the form of radio waves, making it negative and destructive.

The cosmic side of the mind is the sensory activity of creatures in all worlds. It is dominated by visions of the great Gods and Goddesses who, through the Cosmic Mind, fashion the heavens of subtle impressions. Meditation and ritual using form, color and sound help create a positive psychic atmosphere and connect us to the Cosmic Mind.

Composition

The outer mind develops primarily from Rajas, the active energy of consciousness (Chitta).[36] It is built up from the absorbed sensory potentials of sound, touch, sight, taste and smell, along with the emotions and ideas associated with them. As consciousness consists of the gunas, so mind consists of impressions (Tanmatras). The main site of the mind is the head or brain, where the senses predominate, particularly the soft palate which is the central point of all the senses. Its emotional aspect functions through the heart, not the spiritual heart but the physical and vital heart.

Manas constitutes the sheath of mind or Manomaya Kosha. This makes up the subtle or astral body which is the field of our impressions. The subtle body functions in

dream and after-death states. The mind is action predominant[37] and causes us to act in the outer world to establish
our identity as a bodily creature. Through it we take form
and have a function relative to other creatures.

The outer mind adds an additional aspect of water to
the basic air and ether elements of consciousness, and, like
water, has an emotional nature. As such it has qualities in
common with Kapha, the biological water humor. Kapha
people usually have strong emotional natures as well as
sturdy physical bodies, and are well grounded in the realm
of the senses.[38] Similarly, the outer mind relates to Ojas,
the vital essence of water. Ojas is required for developing
and controlling the mind.

Touch and Grasping

Though governing all sense and motor organs, the
mind most corresponds to touch as a sense organ and
grasping (the hands) as a motor organ. Touch is the root of
the lower four sense organs of touch, sight, taste and smell.
It makes sensory impressions intimate and allows us to feel
them personally as pleasure and pain.

Grasping — forming and making, the movement of
the hands — is the main action of the mind, which builds
up our idea of the world. As long as the mind is building
up its world of enjoyment, we must remain trapped in the
cycle of rebirth, ever seeking external happiness. Stopping
this formative action of the mind is the key to going
beyond birth and death.

Energy

The mind is generally personal and is the vehicle for the
ego, but does connect with our genetic background and
species. Through the senses, it connects to our vital nature,

our Pranas, which aligns us with the vital natures of other creatures. As dominated by Rajas, it is easily influenced by the Pranas of ourselves or others, which are similarly the outcome of Rajas or active energy.

The sense mind (Manas) relates to instinct, but governs a more superficial level of instinctual responses than our deeper consciousness (Chitta). The sense mind relates more to the subconscious and our deeper consciousness to the unconscious. Our deeper consciousness governs primal amorphous instincts like sex or the will to live. The mind governs the specific urges of the sense and motor organs, like the desire to speak or walk.

Functions

The outer mind functions to plan, organize and consider, and has the capacity to fashion, make, or imagine. The two main functions of the outer mind, through which it rules over sensation, emotion and thought, are: 1) intention, and 2) imagination[39]

Intention

The mind always has a plan, intention or motivation. It is always constructing something and drawing us into some type of involvement, which tends to be external in orientation. We are always involved in some planned activity, mainly centered around enjoyment for the self or ego through the body and senses. The mind's normal function is to build up our ego world, the realm of achievement and acquisition, for the separate self. Unless we question and control the mind, it will continue to create more involvement and attachments that bring us sorrow. From the mind derive ulterior motives that spoil our actions and remove us from spontaneity. It makes us calculating and self-seeking in all that we do. The result is we can receive no real joy in what we do, which can only come unexpectedly and unsought. To find truth we must go beyond the mind's plans and outer projects.

The mind governs higher intentions as well, including the will to do what is right. Having good intentions and carrying them out is right mental activity. Such good intentions are helping others, surrender to God, and knowing ourselves. The creation of good intentions and good attitudes helps develop the mind properly. These require that we align the mind with our deeper intelligence. When the mind is aligned with our deeper intelligence, it becomes the will to truth and gives the power of renunciation, through which we go beyond self-centered attachments to oneness with all.

Imagination

Imagination is the projection of a possibility, which creates the future. Imagination is part of will, the projection of an intention. We must imagine something as a possibility before we can do it. If we are going to move our hands, for example, we must first imagine doing it. Imagination allows us to project future action, like planning out a trip before taking it. Sensory perception is remembered through imagination. Whatever we have experienced through the senses, the mind can imagine. This ability to reimagine things is the basis for developing knowledge of the world.

In its wrong action, imagination creates wishful thinking that causes illusions. We imagine something to be true when it does not correspond to anything real. We confuse being able to imagine something with actually doing it. This creates many psychological problems. We may imagine many things about ourselves — that we are wise, right or holy — which may have no real basis in our behavior. We confuse our emotional reactions, our personal likes and dislikes, with what things actually are.

The mind governs the dream state, in which our imagination comes freely into play. Mind as the dream state relates to the animal kingdom, which lives in a state of dream or impressions prior to the development of conscious reason.

ADDITIONAL FUNCTIONS

Art and Vision

The outer mind, ruling over expression, governs artistic and creative work. A well-developed sense-mind is necessary for the facility of the motor organs, like the skill of the hands is responsible for the plastic arts. It gives refinement of impressions, particularly when coordinated with intelligence and consciousness. From it comes the creative vision that allows us to create objects of pure form and aesthetic beauty (Sattvic impressions).

For the higher creative function of the mind to develop our enjoyment of subtle sensations, its lower function, which is enjoyment of gross sensations, must be controlled and redirected. The higher function of the mind reveals the subtle senses and psychic abilities that go with them. This includes extrasensory perception (E.S.P.), like seeing or hearing at a distance, and action at a distance (subtle use of the motor organs). All the sensory and motor organs have their subtle counterparts, through which we can experience the subtle world and the occult forces behind the physical world.

Proper Development

The proper development of the mind requires the cultivation of will and character. This depends upon control of the senses, which means taking in the right impressions, and control of emotions, which means separating our emotional reactions from what we actually perceive. Development of artistic capacities, creative vision, occult faculties, or yogic practices involving the chakras are additional aids.

Unfortunately, we have every method of sensory indulgence today through modern technology and the mass media, but no one is taught how to control the senses. Control of the senses seldom enters into our educational system. For this reason our psychological imbalances must increase.

We are always active in life. Our life — from the automatic impulses of the body to the voluntary expressions of the mind — consists of various actions that follow from the will. True will power is not measured by the ability to get what we want but by our ability to transcend desire. Desire is not the result of our free choice. It is a compulsion that comes to us from the external world, a kind of hypnosis. When we give ourselves over to the objects of the senses, they impress the mind, which causes us to want them and to think that our happiness depends upon them. Desire is will that is colored by imagination. It seeks what is external and therefore not really ours.

True will power means that we do what we say and manifest our deeper aspirations in action.[40] Without true will power, it is not possible to gain peace, creativity, or spiritual knowledge. The cultivation of will power gives energy. Various forms of self-discipline, like any voluntary

control of the sensory or motor organs, help develop the
will. We can begin to discipline our physical functions
through fasting or exercise. We can do the same with the
mind. We can fast our minds from wrong impressions or
we can exercise them by repeating a mantra or practicing
concentration.

Character is the ability to control the outer mind and
not be drawn into action by the inertia of external influences. Our senses, with the many stimuli that they bring
in, ever draw us into action. If we act out of the senses, we
lose ourselves and come under the control of the external
world. We lose our consistency of character and merely
reflect the sensations of the moment. Development of
character requires integrity, which is our ability to be true
to our conscience and not follow the impulses of the senses. It depends upon controlling the mind, which means
becoming detached from pleasure and pain, and from sensory desires like food or sex.

The mind is like a lens that opens narrow or wide.
When open wide, it notes many things generally, but little specifically. When narrow, it notes a few things in
detail, but misses the whole. The mind can be turned
within, which requires removing our attention from the
field of the senses. We can train the mind so that it can
open or close at will, allowing us to focus on any particular sensory object or close off from all of them. This
requires control of attention. If we do not train our attention, the mind will follow the urges of the senses according to its conditioning. We will be dominated by external
influences, lose our true self and come under the control of
other people.

Unfortunately we are not trained how to control our
minds, but to give our attention away to various forms of

stimulation and entertainment. This lack of control of the mind and senses allows our energy to go outward, in which it becomes dissipated and fragmented, causing physical and psychological disease. Proper care and usage of the mind, therefore, is essential for our well-being.

9. Ego and Self:
The Quest For Identity

Who Are We?

Who are we? What is the self behind the mind? Sensory impressions rely on our sensory instruments — the eyes, ears and other sense organs. Similarly, emotions and thoughts rely upon our mental instrumentality — the mind. Thought itself is an instrument of knowing. Such instruments require a subject who operates them, just as a microscope or telescope depend upon someone who uses them. The field of thought is a medium through which our subjectivity works. Behind all three layers of consciousness, intelligence, and mind, there is a sense of self that determines their action. All thought rests upon the thought of self.

All of our thoughts refer back to our own identity. All that we do depends upon who we understand ourselves to be. The key to understanding the mind and how it works is to know ourselves. However, who we are is much deeper than what we think, or what society tells us we are. Just as most of our potential consciousness is unknown to us, so most of our potential self-identity, which ultimately includes the entire universe, is not known to us. This ignorance of our true Self is the basis of all our problems in life, whether psychological or spiritual. As we examine the mind and how it works, we are led to the deeper issue of the self and who we are.

Ego — the Separate Self

What human problem can we not easily solve if no one's ego is involved? Ego is the root of all our social and personal problems. Yet what is the ego and how can we deal with it? Is egoism an inevitable part of human nature that cannot be changed, or is there a way to transcend it? Ayurveda tells us that, however deep-seated the ego may be, it is not our true nature. We can go beyond the ego and all its sorrow and conflict.

Ego is called Ahamkara in Sanskrit, which means the "I-process." Ego is a process of self-identification in which we associate our inner being with some outer object or quality. Through it we determine "I am this" or "this is mine." Ego creates the self-image or "I-am-the-body-idea" and results in the sense of separate self. Through it we become isolated and feel different from the world and creatures around us. Ego is the function of consciousness to identify itself with an object, through which we feel ourselves one with a particular body. Only what we have identified as ourselves or as belonging to us, like our family and friends, can we feel deeply about and really bring into our consciousness.

Ego is quite different from our true Self (Atman), which is the pure I am or I-am-that-I-am, the I-in-itself devoid of objectivity. Our true Self stands above all mental and physical forms and conditions, and is ever detached, free and aware. The ego arises from the "I-thought" that stands behind all other thoughts.[41] Whatever thought we have, we must first have the thought of I or self for it to exist. Ego introduces the principle of division, through which consciousness is fragmented and strife becomes possible. It keeps the subjective aspect of our being (self) trapped in some objective form or quality, various bodily sensations or mental states in which there is change and sorrow.

Ego is the primary function of consciousness directed externally. It brings about the entire outward development of consciousness through the mind and body, which are all fragmentations in the field of awareness. Ego affects all the functions of the mind. Everything we do is based upon the self and its motivations. Ego pervades all levels of consciousness and all the bodies of the soul, which require a self-sense for their function. Normally we only know the physical or waking ego, but subtler levels of our nature have their respective egos that allow for their various activities.

The ego concept arises from the atomic nature of the mind. Because we can only focus on one point at a time, we develop the idea of ourselves as a separate center in time and space. By its point-like nature, ego creates a narrow focus or bias, a central blind spot that distorts our vision. Because of this self-sense, all humans have an inherent feeling of pride. We like to think that we or what we identify with — our religion, country, race, class, or family — is the best or the only valid one. This process of pride causes us to look down on others and creates conflict.

Ego and the Functions of the Mind

Ego arises from a failure of intelligence (Buddhi). It is a misjudgment or error in our perceptual process. The most important function of intelligence is to ascertain the nature of the self. Self-determination is the most primary of all determinations. First we must know who we are before we can know what the world is or what we should do. Ego arises when we fail to discern our true Self, which is pure awareness, and mistake it for the body, which is no more than an object.

However, once intelligence makes the mistake of the ego, the ego distorts intelligence, which then serves to rationalize it. We use our intelligence to further the ego's goals of accumulation and achievement in the external world, and lose track of our inner goal, which is to know our real nature. This ego of intelligence is the hardest ego to overcome because it is so primary a misconception. Some thinkers regard Buddhi or intelligence as the Self.[42] This is a mistake, because the Self transcends all movements of thought. However, since intelligence is close to the Self, it can lead us gradually to it.

Our deeper consciousness (Chitta) precedes the manifest ego but itself contains a rudimentary or latent ego. As a part of matter (Prakriti), consciousness has an inertia to take form that develops through the ego. Ego uses our deeper consciousness to cling to life and to sustain its experience. The rudimentary ego hidden in our deeper consciousness gradually evolves into all the diversification of the mind-body complex.

From ego arises the outer mind (Manas), senses and body, through which we experience our separate existence. The sense-mind, by its outward propensity, is naturally under the sway of the ego, and only with difficulty can be brought under the control of true intelligence. Ego operates through the mind to acquire sensations that allow it to expand and feel good about itself. The ultimate crystallization of the ego is the physical body, in which we experience ourselves as completely separate from other creatures.

Whatever function occurs in consciousness, an ego is automatically posited as part of its boundary. Each emotion projects a kind of ego. For example, the ego of anger is very different from the ego of love. We run into problems in our behavior when the ego of our emotions drives us to actions that we later regret.

Because ego is inherently limited and isolating, it must bring unhappiness. It causes us to identify with some things and not with others. When we lose those objects we have identified with, we must feel pain. When we contact what we are not identified with, what we regard as alien to ourselves, we also experience pain.

Ego and Perception

Ego arises automatically during the perceptual process. As the thought of I underlies all thoughts, so the sensation of I underlies all impressions. The sense-mind (Manas) provides a series of sensory impressions, for which the body is the main focus and instrument. The ego inherent in body-consciousness colors all these. Ego appropriates impressions, such as "I like this" or "I do not like that," "I love this," or "I hate that." Similarly, ego appropriates intelligence and uses it to justify its own reactions. Its logic is that "I must be right" or "I must be good." Ego stops intelligence from perceiving the truth and instead imposes its own opinion as truth.

The ego cannot appropriate our deeper consciousness (Chitta), but it can narrow and distort it. We can only become aware of that part of our consciousness acceptable to the ego. Ego is our most basic subconscious reaction that keeps the greater field of consciousness suppressed. We must learn to observe our perceptual process to transcend the ego. This requires that our deeper consciousness is in a state of peace and that our intelligence functions objectively. The ego as a form of ignorance (Tamas) and distraction (Rajas) becomes reduced as we no longer provide the environment in which it can flourish.

Cosmic Aspect of Ego

Each individual creature must have some sort of ego. Ego exists even in insects and rocks. It is ego that allows for the gross elements and inanimate world to come into being. The inanimate creation is pure ego, so contracted that it does not allow any action of the vital force or senses, which require consciousness of the external world.

Ego exists as a cosmic principle. From it the root ideals and archetypes of creation (which are inherent in Cosmic Intelligence) can be diversified. Ego is responsible for the creation of the different objects, creatures and worlds. From it the gross and subtle elements arise. We can perceive higher cosmic states of ego once we expand our sense of self into the deeper levels of consciousness. We can move from being identified with our body to being identified with our family, country, world, and universe — and ultimately to being one with all beings.

Composition

Ego is the seed of Tamas (darkness) or the Tamasic side of consciousness (Chitta). It corresponds to the earth element or the heavy matters in consciousness. Ego develops from ignorance, not knowing our true nature as pure Consciousness. It is the source of attraction, repulsion and attachment, the emotional afflictions that bring pain and sorrow. It puts us under the rule of all duality, the ups and downs of our emotional experience.

As the power of ignorance, ego relates to the mineral kingdom in which no sensitivity has developed. The ego is the inertia of the rock — matter asserting its existence apart from the spirit. As isolation and fragmentation, it is the source of decay, disease and death. Transcending the ego is the basic evolutionary movement of life, through

which we form associations and seek to know the greater
universe in which we live.

Energy

Ego relates to the heavy matters that accumulate in our
consciousness and so has an energy of inertia (Tamas). It
relates to Apana Vayu or the downward moving Prana that
brings about disease and decay. Ego drives us to fragmentation and ultimately to self-destruction, unless we learn
how to control it. Its energy is negative, or entropy, and
leads to eventual loss of energy.

Function

The ego allows us to identify with and feel one with
things. Through it we build up a self-identity based upon
the objects and conditions we have accepted as our own. It
functions in two ways: 1) self-sense, and 2) mine-ness.[43]

Self-sense is the sense of owning a body, through which
we know the body as I or me. Self-sense also expropriates
the mind, identifying with its various thoughts, emotions
and sensations, such as "I am wise" or "I am happy." Mine-
ness is the sense of owning external objects, which we
accumulate around our bodily existence. Through it we
feel that particular objects, like our house, money, or job,
belong to us. Mine-ness depends upon and follows from
self-sense. Through mineness, the ego establishes its terri-
tory and grows and expands in the outer world. As long as
we have a sense of ownership or possession of anything, we
are caught in the ego and its bonds.

The ego, like the sense-mind, has an outgoing energy,
but while the mind seeks enjoyment in the realm of the
senses, the ego seeks to embody itself in a material form.
The ego's identification of the self with a body sets in
motion the entire cycle of rebirth.

On the positive side, ego as self-sense provides a focus of mind. It helps consciousness differentiate who we are from the external nature. It causes us to evolve a personal and social existence apart from the instinctual and animal realm. But ego is not the final goal of Nature's evolution, nor does it represent who we really are. Ego is the point of transition between the material and spiritual evolution. It is an intermediate phase between an outward-directed mentality under the control of Nature, and an inward-directed mind in harmony with the Spirit.

The Soul — Our Divine Individuality

Ego is our sense of transient identity, that we are the creature of a particular life or body. The soul, on the other hand, is the sense that we are an immortal conscious being, an individualized portion of Divinity. This soul is called Jiva in Sanskrit, the life-principle, because it is the source of all our vitality and energy, both physical and mental. It is also called Jivatman, the individual or living (Jiva) Self (Atman). It is our individual portion of the Divine Self through which we have the sense of "I am." The individual soul is the higher self-sense behind our individual existence, our true individuality.

The soul is the entity behind the causal body, composed of our various karmas, that persists throughout the entire cycle of rebirth. As a soul we recognize ourselves as immortal conscious beings, born in various bodies, seeking Self-realization and liberation. The soul leads us back to unity while the ego drives us into division and multiplicity.

We are usually not conscious of the soul or reincarnating entity within us. Nevertheless it creates and sustains all that we do. The soul exists everywhere in Nature, giving life and sustaining form in all things. The soul is latent in the elemental kingdom. It sleeps in the plants, dreams in animals, wakes in human beings, and becomes fully conscious of itself in Self-realized sages.

Most of us experience the soul (deep feeling) only with other human beings, with the feeling of love. We do it to some extent with animals, particularly pets. It is possible to communicate with the soul in plants and the soul in the elements as well. We can feel our soul in all existence.

The cosmic counterpart of the soul is God (Ishvara), the creator of the universe, who is the Lord of all souls and the dispenser of the fruits of all karmas. As our self-sense becomes universalized, we can experience the reality of God within our minds and commune with the Creator. We feel ourselves as servants or workers for God, following His will, which is for the full unfoldment of consciousness in the universe.

Energy

The soul controls all our positive energy, creativity and vitality. It sustains the master Prana behind our deeper consciousness (Chitta). All that was said relative to this applies here as well.

Composition

The soul (Jiva) is the entity inherent in our deeper consciousness (Chitta) as its awakened or Sattvic function. For this reason, the soul is not always differentiated from Chitta in its pure form or from the awakened intelligence (Buddhi), both of which function through Sattva. The purification of Chitta and the awakening of intelligence come about through the soul coming forth and taking charge of our existence.

The soul (Jiva) becomes conscious through the pure

Sattva developed in our various lives. Through it, the causal Prana (vital force) arises by which we become alive and animate. The soul is the source of life (Prana), love (Chitta) and light (Buddhi), which are its three main powers. Because of it we wish to live forever, to be perfectly happy, and to know absolute truth.

Functions

The soul works through the power of identification but, unlike the ego, it expands its field of identification to include all of which it is aware. It has two main functions: 1) Self-knowledge, and 2) Surrender to God.

The soul's knowledge is Self-knowledge — knowledge of our true nature as Pure Consciousness. This allows us to find unity with all that we perceive and opens up all the secrets of the universe to us. Its main action is surrender to God (Ishvara-pranidhana) and following the Divine will. The higher functions of consciousness and intelligence, like samadhi and intuition, function through it. Through the individual Self, both consciousness and intelligence get activated, causing knowledge of truth, immortality and infinity.[44]

To really enter the spiritual path, we must become conscious of ourselves on a soul level. This requires getting to the real soul awareness that lies hidden in our deeper consciousness (Chitta). The soul comes forward when we set aside our sense of bodily identity and recognize ourselves as an individualized portion of Divinity. When the soul comes forth, we set aside our transient ego goals and organize our lives toward our eternal goal of God-realization. The soul is the most subtle form of ego or individuality, through which we can go beyond the ego.

The Soul and Healing

Getting to the level of the soul is the key to all forms of healing. The soul is the great healer because it is one with both God and Nature and carries all their powers and grace. It is not so much that we need to heal our souls as that we have to become aware of our souls. Becoming aware of our soul is the deepest healing possible, not only for the soul but also for the mind. The awareness of the soul releases all the healing powers inherent within us.

The word soul, however, can have many meanings, according to different thinkers. Some call soul our emotional nature. Others see it as connected to some heavenly realm that is our ultimate goal, like an angel. The Vedic idea of the soul (Jiva), however, is the first individualized portion of consciousness. The true soul is not an emotional belief, but a state of higher awareness beyond all forms and preconceptions. It does not belong to any particular religion and is not in need of salvation. Rather, the soul itself leads to all redemption and transformation because it transcends the limitations of the ego, mind and body.

The Supreme Self — Our Divine Nature

The mind is not the source of consciousness or awareness. Any conditioned consciousness — consciousness dependent upon thought, emotion or sensation — is not true consciousness at all. It is like a light reflected in a mirror, not the true source of the light. True consciousness is beyond all objects and qualities, and not dependent upon any physical, sensory or mental instrumentality. This pure consciousness is our true Self. In our unconditioned Self we are one with all beings. This is the Supreme Self (Paramatman) of Vedanta, the supreme Vedic philosophy behind Ayurveda.[45]

The Supreme Self exists beyond both God and the individual soul. It transcends all beings, all worlds, and all three gunas. While conditioned consciousness (Chitta) is composed of thoughts, the true Self is thought-free awareness (Chit). The Self is the real light that illumines the modifications of the mind and is never affected by them. It is the unity behind both the soul and God, which includes all the world of Nature in the formless Absolute. It is the immutable peace at the core of the mind, through which we immediately transcend all psychological problems.

Through setting aside the ego and awakening our soul (Jiva), we bring ourselves gradually into contact with this higher Self. Any contact with our true Self lifts us beyond all human and creaturely problems. Because the purpose of this book is more psychological, we will not examine this Self in depth. This occurs in the teaching of Vedanta.[46] To calm psychological disturbances, it is often enough to restore the proper usage of the conditioned mind. Yet to go beyond all sorrow we must know our true Self, and any real healing of the mind benefits from even the slightest contact with our true nature.

All the methods given in this book for psychological healing also aid in the higher goal of Self-realization. Removing negative conditioning from the mind is necessary for both psychological harmony and for Self-realization. The difference is that, to perceive our true Self, a much deeper level of deconditioning has to be achieved than is necessary for resolving our psychological problems, like fear, anger or depression. The Yogi's concern is developing consciousness to create the appropriate vessel for the perception of the Self, which is always present but obscured by our shifting thoughts. The Ayurvedic physician's concern is developing consciousness to counter our ordinary human problems. Purification of consciousness[47] is common to both. It is the most important thing both for mental health and for spiritual growth.

The Self and Functions of the Mind

The three main layers of the mind — consciousness, intelligence and sense-mind — function between ego, or false self, on one side and the true Self on the other. Their actions vary according to the direction in which they are oriented. Directed toward the Self, their higher functions emerge. Directed toward the ego and external world, their higher potential remains latent and they conflict with one another.

Consciousness (Chitta) is closer to the Self, while the sense-mind (Manas) is closer to the ego. Intelligence (Buddhi), which is placed between them, is the key factor in how we orient our awareness. Because of its capacity for decisive perception, intelligence has a power of spiritual transformation greater than either the sense-mind or deeper consciousness. It can empty consciousness of its conditioning and control the sense-mind. It can question the ego and discriminate between the lower and the higher Self.

True intelligence discerns our higher self-identity that leads to our true nature. This is the identity of consciousness, not the self-image or ego which depends for its being upon an object or quality. The soul works through the higher aspect of intelligence, which is its development of the mental field according to the light of truth. The true Self awakens when we bring our awareness to the field of consciousness as a whole by the upward and inward movement of intelligence. Otherwise dominated by the downward and outward movement of the sense-mind, we become trapped in the forces of the external world, which leads to both ignorance and sorrow.

Layers of Consciousness and Psychological Disease

Manas is the outer layer of consciousness through which we are involved with the events of the moment. Buddhi is the middle layer of consciousness that allows us to observe both what is happening in the immediate sense and the long term. Chitta is the deeper layer of consciousness that holds long-term patterns.

When we learn something new, like tying our shoes, it is at first a process of Manas, through which we perform the action working with the senses. Buddhi is involved as the director of the action, through which we develop our skill in performing it. Once what we have learned becomes second nature, it becomes a function of Chitta. We tie our shoes automatically without any deliberation through this power of Chitta. In the ordinary person, we can divide the layers of consciousness accordingly:

Chitta — unconscious, but also potential higher consciousness

Manas — subconscious

Buddhi — conscious

Ahamkara — self-conscious

Chitta is the total potential field of conditioned consciousness (the field of thought). Manas contains all sensory reactions which are largely subliminal. In this regard, Manas and Chitta are close together and what we take in through the senses automatically influences the unconscious. Only Buddhi is the aware part of consciousness. It can divide Chitta from Manas so that our sensory responses do not condition us at a deeper level. Ahamkara is self-consciousness or ego that makes us vulnerable to external influences. The Atman witnesses and transcends all these functions and is contacted through the higher function of the Buddhi.

In the disease process, the Doshas or disease-causing factors are the wrong functioning of mind and intelligence, which occurs through the ego. The ego introduces Rajas and Tamas, the mental Doshas, into the mental field in the form of negative thoughts, emotions and impressions. It makes us use our senses, emotion and intellect for selfish enjoyment rather than for developing a higher consciousness. Wrong functioning of intelligence (Buddhi) is the main disease-causing factor because it regulates how we use the mind and senses.

Chitta is the aspect of the mind that is damaged by these disease-causing factors. Like the tissues of the body damaged by wrong use of the sense organs and poor digestion, consciousness is the substance of the mind damaged by wrong mental activity. For treating the mind, we must eliminate these mental toxins and also repair the mental substance (consciousness).[48]

Functions of the Mind

While each function of the mind has its natural qualities (gunas), it can be altered by an admixture of other gunas. Understanding the gunas of the mind and changing them from Tamas to Sattva is the key to mental health and spiritual development. The whole of spiritual development and psychological healing consists of moving from Tamasic to Sattvic living.[49]

We all go through various gunic phases in our daily activity. When we are asleep or mentally dull, we are in a Tamasic mode. When we are awake and perceptive, we are in a Sattvic mode. When we are active or distracted, we are in a Rajasic mode. Generally what we do in a Tamasic or Rajasic mode — something ignorant, unfeeling or foolish (Tamas) or something aggressive, agitated or impulsive (Rajasic) — we regret while in a Sattvic (peaceful) mode. Yet we should not get discouraged. Even an enlightened person can have Tamasic moments when he may do something that he may later regret. Our karma is not determined by our Tamasic moments only, but by all three gunas at play within our mental field.

Look at the play of these three gunas in your mental condition. For example, some people will be more Sattvic in the morning and turn dull and Tamasic in the evening. Others will be dull and Tamasic in the morning but Sattvic in the evening. Some people are more active or Rajasic in the morning, others in the evening. Generally Sattva should prevail more in the morning and evening, with Rajas developing more midday and Tamas only during sleep.

Note how your environment and associations affect you. Around Sattvic (spiritual) people and situations you will feel Sattvic. Around Tamasic (dull) people and situations you will feel dull and depressed. Around Rajasic (disturbed) people and situations you will feel agitated. See how your life is developing. Are you becoming more Sattvic (spiritual), Rajasic (busy) or Tamasic (dull)?

FUNCTIONS OF THE MIND

	SATTVA	RAJAS	TAMAS
Consciousness (Chitta)	inner peace, selfless love, faith, joy, devotion, compassion, receptivity, clarity, good intuition, deep understanding, detachment, fearlessness, inner silence, clear memory, calm sleep, right relationships	emotional disturbances, overactive imagination, uncontrolled thoughts, worry, discontent, desire, irritability, anger, distorted memory, disturbed sleep, turbulent relationships	deep-seated emotional blockages & attachments, trapped in past patterns & memories, addictions, worry, phobias, fear, anxiety, depression, hatred, excessive sleep, wrong relationships
Intelligence (Buddhi)	discrimination between the eternal & the transient, clear perception, strong ethics, tolerance, non-violence, truthfulness, honesty, clarity, cleanliness	critical mind, judgmental, opinionated, self-righteous, assertive, narrow-minded, distorted perception, believes in the reality of the outer world or in particular names & forms as truth	lack of intelligence, lack of perception, deep prejudices, lack of conscience or ethics, dishonesty, delusions, believes in the reality of one's own opinions
Mind (Manas)	good self-control, control of senses, control of sexual desire, ability to endure pain, ability to withstand the elements (heat & cold), detachment from the body, does what one says	strong sensate nature, strong sexual nature, many desires, aggressive, assertive, competitive, willful, overly active imagination, disturbed dreams, willful, calculating	lazy, lacking self-control, easily influenced by others, aimless thinking, daydreaming, unable to endure pain, caught up in violent sensations, many habits & addictions, easily influenced, taking of drugs, dissipation
Ego (Ahamkara)	spiritual idea of self, selflessness, surrender, devotion, self-knowledge, concern for others, respect for all creatures, compassion	ambitious, assertive, achievement-oriented, willful, arrogant, vain, self-promoting, manipulative, strong identifications (as with family, country, religion)	negative idea of self, fearful, slavish, dependent, dishonest, fear, identified mainly with one's own body

How to Properly Develop the Functions of the Mind

Chitta	Pranayama, mantra, meditation on infinite space or the void, concentration and mindfulness techniques, Samadhi, devotion (Bhakti Yoga) and knowledge (Jnana Yoga) combined, right beliefs, receptivity, clarity, faith, love, peace, joy, communion, right associations, satsang (spiritual communion)
Buddhi	Concentration, meditation, Self-inquiry, mantra, meditation, contemplation of universal truths, yoga of knowledge (Jnana Yoga), self-examination, development of conscience and ethics, right reasoning, self-discipline, developing Tejas (inner fire)
Manas	Devotion (particularly using a particular form or image), self-discipline (like fasting), control of sexual energy, mantra, meditation on inner light and sound, visualization, work, service, Yoga of Devotion (Bhakti Yoga), Ojas enhancement therapies, right intake of impressions, right diet, practice of patience, development of character, will-power and control of senses
Ahamkara	Spiritual aspiration, devotion to God, selfless service, self-discipline, self-inquiry, self-observation, right association

Exercises in Consciousness

The following are some simple exercises in consciousness to help you understand the different levels of your mind and how they are working to make your life more creative and aware or more constricted and asleep.

Taking an Inventory of Your Consciousness

Examine the weight of your life experience: the substances and energies you have taken into yourself through your habitual actions and expressions. Look at the quality of your food, impressions, and associations, the emotions you have most frequently, the thoughts and beliefs which motivate you. See what you hold most dear, what abides most deeply in your heart, what you most give your attention to.

On one side, place all your negative life activities — negative emotions (anger, lust, fear, ambition, violence), pursuit of pleasure, desire, and selfishness. On the other side, place all your positive life activities — meditation, prayer, spiritual study, good works, social service, and so on. Note the balance. Your consciousness is the storehouse of all this experience. Its nature depends upon the predominance of your mental activity, particularly at a heart level.

Another way to do this is to examine your spontaneous and automatic reactions, to see what your programming is. Note your immediate reactions to situations, particularly those in which you are taken off guard, or are in some way threatened. Note also your consciousness during habitual states like sleeping, eating, entertainment and other mechanical activities, when you are not engaged in any specific mental activity. This underlying inertia of the mind is your consciousness (Chitta).

Examining Your Intelligence

See where your sense of discrimination is most developed, whether it is food, movies, sex, sports, scientific information, politics, art, philosophy, or spiritual knowledge. See where your intelligence has its greatest refinement, clarity and depth. See if you have cultivated an outer sense of discrimination, developing opinions about people or situations, or an inner sense, learning to discern the inner truth or reality of things.

Note where your sense of discrimination naturally goes, what you are most commonly calculating. Note where you most exercise your sense of choice, value and judgment. Through this process you can understand the nature of your intelligence and how it is likely to develop.

Examining the Outer Mind and Senses

Observe how you use your senses, which senses you use most and in what manner. See to what extent sensory influences dominate you. How do you relate to audio, tactile, visual and other sensations? To what degree can you control your mind's attention and not be distracted by sensory influences. What sensations most attract and bind your mind? What mental and emotional impressions and influences most affect you through the senses (fear, anger, desire, love, or hate). See what mental impressions and information most affects you. See how your senses control you and dominate your attention.

Do the same in regard to the motor organs. See what control you have over your vocal organs, hands, feet, reproductive and eliminatory organs. Can you turn off their activities and detach yourself from their urges or are you under their power? These mental exercises provide a good measure of how much you are in control of the mind or how much your mind controls you.

Examining the Ego

See what you most identify with in life — occupation, family, friends, property, country, religion and so on. See how closely you identify with your body, senses, opinions, emotions and ideas. Examine what you most fear losing and what you are most trying to gain: pleasure, wealth, power, name, fame and so on. Imagine that you are dying today and have to let everything go. See how difficult this may be and what most holds you to this world.

Once we have examined all our mental functions, we can see how our life is likely to develop. We can determine how susceptible we may be not only to psychological problems but to sorrow in general. Just as you keep track of your health through regular physical examinations, keep track of your psychological condition through regular mental examinations.

The Chakras

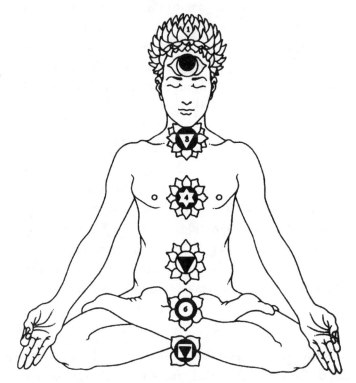

1. HEAD CENTER
Consciousness-Space
Causal Sound
Causal Prana
Om

2. THIRD EYE
Mind-Space
Sublte Sound
Subtle Prana
Ksham

3. THROAT CENTER
Ether
Sound
Vata
Ham

4. HEART CENTER
Air
Touch
Vata
Yam

5. NAVEL CENTER
Fire
Sight
Pitta
Ram

6. SEX CENTER
Water
Taste
Kapha
Vam

7. ROOT CENTER
Earth
Smell
Kapha
Lam

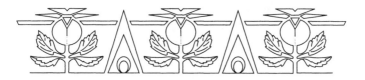

Part III

AYURVEDIC THERAPIES FOR THE MIND

Ayurvedic therapies are multifaceted for improving mental well-being and promoting spiritual growth. Those introduced here are primarily of a self-help nature, but may require additional guidance to employ them optimally. The section begins with Ayurvedic counseling methods and the Ayurvedic view of treating the different aspects of the mind. Then it discusses the Ayurvedic science of impressions and how we can alter them to improve our mental function.

Specific chapters follow on outer treatment modalities like diet and herbs, and inner methods, mainly sensory techniques of colors, gems and aromas, leading to mantra, which is the most important Ayurvedic tool for changing our consciousness. As these treatment methods are diverse, this is the longest section of the book, but also perhaps the most practical and useful.

10. Ayurvedic Counseling and Behavioral Modification

Communication is the basis of who we are and what we seek to become. We do not exist in isolation, nor can we grow apart from the cultural matrix that sustains us. The mind itself is primarily a communication device, not only for relating outwardly to other people, but relating inwardly to the spiritual forces of the universe. This importance of communication extends into the sphere of healing as well.

Counseling is probably the most important instrument of psychological treatment. However, from the Ayurvedic standpoint, it should not be merely talk or discussion but a prescription for action. Counseling should examine the causes of psychological imbalances and indicate how to correct them. No one will continue in a pattern that he or she knows is harmful, but we must truly understand the harmful nature of our behavior to be willing to change. Counseling should be a learning process in which the client comes to understand the different aspects of his or her nature and how to modify these for optimal well-being.

In this chapter we will discuss the Ayurvedic counseling approach that forms the background for Ayurvedic psychological therapies. We will look into the issues that arise in counseling through the different Ayurvedic constitutional types. Ayurvedic counseling deals in four primary areas:

1) Physical factors — diet, herbs and exercise;

2) Psychological factors — impressions, emotions, thought;

3) Social factors — work, recreation, relationship; and

4) Spiritual factors — yoga and meditation.

Physical and psychological imbalances reinforce each other, with diet and exercise reflecting our state of mind and its fluctuations. Psychological imbalances involve social and personal problems, like career and relationship difficulties. Spiritual factors are the ultimate sources of any mental distress because only our higher consciousness has the power to bring peace to the mind, which is inherently changing and unstable. Therefore, Ayurvedic psychology deals with four levels of treatment:

1. Biological humors — Balancing Vata, Pitta and Kapha;

2. Vital essences — Strengthening Prana, Tejas and Ojas, the master forms of Vata, Pitta and Kapha;

3. Impressions — Harmonizing the mind and senses; and

4. Consciousness — Promoting the correct functions of consciousness.

Ayurveda first works on balancing the biological humors through appropriate physical remedial methods of diet, herbs, and exercise. Typical books on Ayurveda focus on this level. We will examine these outer treatment methods of Ayurveda in a subsequent chapter, particularly as they affect psychological conditions. Second, Ayurveda works to improve our vital energy through Pranayama and related practices. The section on Prana, Tejas and Ojas discusses this level and it is mentioned occasionally throughout the book.

Third, Ayurveda works on the mind and senses to promote the right intake of impressions through various sensory therapies. In the following chapters, we will examine these sensory therapies, particularly aromas and colors. Fourth, Ayurveda works to increase Sattva in our consciousness through spiritual living principles, mantra and meditation. This we will examine in the chapters on Mantra, Spiritual Therapies and the Eightfold Method of Yoga.

Ayurvedic counseling is very practical and involves various prescriptions for changing how we live. Meeting with an Ayurvedic counselor involves reviewing the results of implementing these prescriptions, and is done in a consistent step-by-step manner. Ayurvedic counseling is educational in nature. The therapist helps the client learn how the mind and body work so that we can use them properly. The patient is a student. Therapy is a learning process. Ayurveda looks upon someone suffering from a psychological problem not as a bad or disturbed person, but as someone who does not understand how to use the mind properly.

Right Association — a Key to Mental Health

Who we are psychologically is a result of how we interact with our environment. If you want to see what you are, look at the people you feel closest to and with whom you spend the most time. The mind is built up by the impressions taken in through the senses, most important of which are those that come from our social interactions. Whatever impressions we take in become more powerful when shared with other people, who give them emotional power.

The mind itself, down to the deepest unconscious, is a social entity and follows a collective pattern. It is made up of thought, conditioned by the language used in the social context of our lives. The mind reflects our interactions with other people, starting with our parents. The mind is the record of our associations, which includes not only human beings but all life to which we are related. Our deeper consciousness (Chitta) itself is determined by the nature of our associations, which create the most powerful impulses (Samskaras) that we have to deal with. If we go to the core of our hearts, it is our closest relationships that most determine who we are.

Ayurvedic psychology emphasizes right association to ensure psychological well-being. We should always be careful to keep ourselves in the right company. We should associate with those individuals who elevate us, who bring peace and keep our minds cool and calm. We should keep ourselves distant from those who drag us down, who agitate and overheat our minds and nerves. We must be most careful about who we associate with on an intimate level.

We should seek the good and strive to be in the company of the wise. Such are spiritual teachers, true friends, the beauty of nature, great art, and wisdom teachings. Of course, it is not always possible to remain in the physical company of spiritually elevating people. They are not always easy to find or to gain time with. However, we can always keep them in our minds and hearts. We can attune ourselves with their thoughts and deeds. In turn, we ourselves should strive to have a beneficial influence on others, projecting helpful attitudes and good thoughts toward the entire universe.

Healing the mind involves healing how we relate to the world. It means establishing a society or group of friends that draws us upward. This is the basis of real counseling. The counselor should provide the client with a deeper level of association that does not reinforce their problems, but, on the contrary, provides a space for their problems to be released. Ideally, a true therapist should not be a doctor in the distance, but a spiritual friend and well-wisher. Therapy should be the beginning of communion, what is called in Sanskrit Satsanga, the company of those sincerely seeking truth.

However, better than going to a therapist is frequenting the company of spiritually elevating people. In their company, our psychological problems, which come from our material involvement, naturally get resolved. The mere presence of such wise people cools and calms the mind and heart. Lack of spiritual company is a main cause of psychological unrest and the only cure is to find such association.

Discussing our problems, particularly with someone we respect, is always of great help. It takes us beyond the personal nature of our problems to the greater and universal issues of life. Communication itself is much of the benefit of psychotherapy — drawing us into a relationship that allows our problems to be discussed. Communication breaks down the walls of isolation in which we suffer and helps us look at ourselves in a new light, allowing old patterns of constriction to be broken down and discarded.

A true spiritual teacher helps us know who we are in our inner consciousness, as apart from our ordinary identification with the mind-body complex. Such a person is the ultimate psychologist. However, a spiritual teacher may not be interested in functioning as a psychologist or a doctor in the ordinary sense, helping us with our personal worries, woes, aches and pains. The role of the spiritual teacher is to guide us to higher states of consciousness, not merely to help us resolve our ordinary problems. This may involve teaching us to be detached from both our psychological and physical sufferings, which must always exist in this transient world.

A therapist, on the other hand, must recognize the limits of what he or she can do. Therapists should not play guru, but direct their clients toward genuine spiritual teachers. Spiritual guidance is much more than psychology in the ordinary sense, though true psychology should lead to spirituality. Spirituality requires that we go beyond the mind and its opinions, not merely that we are happy with our state of mind.

Psychological Disorders and the Biological Humors

Psychological disorders, like physical ones, reflect imbalances of the three biological humors. Health problems, whether physical or mental, are not merely personal problems, but energetic problems in the mind-body complex. They are not so much personal or moral failings as an inability to harmonize the forces within us.

Vata (Air) Type

Psychological disturbances occur with greater frequency when Vata is too high, which, as the nervous force, easily affects the mind. Like Vata, the mind is composed of the air and ether elements. Vata's excess of air causes instability and agitation in the mind, which results in excessive thinking or worrying and makes our problems appear worse than they really are. The mind becomes overly sensitive, excessively reactive, and we take things too personally. We are prone to premature or inappropriate action that may aggravate our problems.

High Vata, as excess ether, makes us ungrounded, spaced-out and unrealistic. We may have various wrong imaginations, hallucinations or delusions, like hearing voices. Our connection with the physical body and with physical reality becomes weakened. We live in our thoughts, which we may confuse with perception. Our life-force gets dispersed by the excess activity of the mind. We lose contact with other people and cannot heed their advice.

High Vata in the mind manifests as fear, alienation, anxiety and possible nervous breakdown. There is insomnia, tremors, palpitations, unrest and rapid shifts of mood. Insanity of the manic depressive type, or schizophrenia, is an extreme Vata imbalance.

There are many factors that can disturb Vata and create possible psychological problems. Disturbing sensations are hard for Vatas to handle, particularly too much exposure to the mass media, loud music or noise. Drugs and stimulants easily derange them. Insufficient food or irregular eating also weakens and upsets them mentally. Excessive or unnatural sexual activity quickly drains their often low energy. Stress, fear and anxiety affect them emotionally because they lack calm and endurance. Violence and trauma leaves them hurt and withdrawn. Neglect or abuse as a child creates a predisposition for a Vata-deranged psychology.

Pitta (Fire) Type

Psychological disturbances are moderate in Pitta types. They usually have strong self-control but can be self-centered and antisocial. The fire and heat of Pitta cause the mind to be narrow and contentious, fighting either with others or with themselves. Pitta psychological disorders are typically due to too much aggression or hostility. Typical Pitta is the overly critical type who finds fault with everyone, blames other people for everything, sees enemies everywhere, is always on guard and ready for a fight.

High Pitta in the mind causes agitation, irritation, anger, and possible violence. The overheated body and mind seek release in venting the built-up tension. Pitta types can become domineering, authoritarian or fanatic. When disturbed they may have paranoid delusions, delusions of grandeur, or can become psychotic.

Pitta in the mind becomes too high by various factors that increase heat. Strong and bright colors and sensations quickly irritate them. Exposure to violence and aggression increases the same attitudes within them. Dietary factors like overly hot or spicy food disturb their minds. Sexual frustration, excessive anger and ambition, and related emotional factors take their toll. Too competitive an education or too much conflict in childhood are additional factors.

Kapha (Water) Type

Kapha people have the least amount of psychological problems and are the least likely to express them or to resort to antisocial behavior. Kapha disturbs the mind by blocking the channels and clouding the senses. High Kapha (mucus and water) generally causes mental dullness, congestion and poor perception.

Kapha psychological unrest involves attachment and lack of motivation leading to depression, sorrow, and clinging. The mind may be incapable of abstract, objective or impersonal thinking. There is a lack of drive and motivation along with passivity and dependency. We want to remain a child and be taken care of. We become preoccupied with what others think about us. We lack the proper self-image and passively reflect our immediate environment. Such people often end up being taken care of by others and are unable to function on their own.

However, stronger Kapha types can suffer from greed and possessiveness, which renders the mind heavy, dull and depressed. They want to own and control everything and look upon people as their property as well. Once they lose control or ownership, they become psychologically unstable.

Kapha emotional disturbances result from excess pleasure, enjoyment, or attachment in life. Lifestyle factors like too much sleep, sleep during the day, or lack of exercise contribute to these. Kapha-aggravating diet, like too much sugar or oily food, is another factor. Emotional problems combine with Kapha physical conditions like overweight and congestion. Educational factors include being overly indulged as a child or emotionally smothered by parents.

Ayurvedic Counseling Profiles

The constitutional types of Ayurveda are the basis of all Ayurvedic counseling. They are useful for understanding the different types of people and their interactions that can occur. They are an extension of the psychological profiles of the biological humors and their characteristic psychological disorders. Again, these are general profiles and should not be taken rigidly.

Vata

Vata types are nervous, anxious or afraid. They are often worried, upset or distracted, even if there is no real problem in their lives. They may be hesitant and insecure, which they may exhibit by moving around or fidgeting.

Under the influence of air or wind they find it difficult to settle down or be at ease. They have many doubts about themselves and their ability to get well or about any treatment and its ability to help them.

Sometimes they are over-enthusiastic and excited when starting a therapy, but this seldom lasts and may be followed by quickly quitting or getting frustrated. They expect too much and want immediate results. They may look to the therapist to heal them magically and when this does not occur they get disappointed or seek to change therapists. They are often ungrounded and hard to pin down. They have to become realistic about their condition and the effort required to correct it. They must come back to earth about themselves and their behavior.

Vata types often have a negative attitude about themselves. They will have more worries and negative imaginations about their disease condition than it merits. They are commonly hypochondriacs. They need to calm their minds and hearts as part of any treatment. They are often looking for attention and sympathy more than developing their own understanding. They are happy to receive advice but not consistent in following it. They require much time and patience to really change. Their condition will fluctuate, sometimes dramatically, along with their thoughts. Slow steady development with peace of mind is what they should aim for.

They seek comfort and require a lot of assurance, but this does not always make them feel secure. They like to talk at length about their problems but this may not be of great help. They do best if they try a few practical things to improve their condition and implement these in a consistent manner. This fosters a realistic attitude about dealing with their condition and does not feed their excessive mental activity.

Vata types can be so caught up in their problems that they do not take the time to do something about them. They can be looking so hard for external support that they do not do the things that allow them to take control of their own lives. They need to emphasize action rather than thought, steady application rather than looking for results.

They need to follow a clear and comprehensive life-regimen to bring stability to their minds, calm their agitated life-force, and cushion their sensitive hearts. The rule is to treat them like a flower. They easily feel frightened and are prone to withdraw if approached forcefully. They must be approached with warmth, calm and determination and made to feel the support of others, yet without making them dependent.

Pitta

Pitta types think that they already know who they are and what they are doing. If they have problems, they usually have someone or something to blame, or attribute their problems to not being able to achieve their goals. They are most disturbed by conflict with other people, which they often exaggerate or exacerbate. The drama of interpersonal struggle colors their minds and emotions. These conflicts can be internalized and result in self-conflict. Pitta types are prone to be at war with themselves and easily internalize external conflicts.

Having a fiery nature, they tend to be aggressive, critical, sometimes contentious, and can be destructive. They may question the qualifications of their therapists. They are the most likely of the different types to tell the therapist what he or she should do for them. They are the most likely to respond with anger or criticism if the treatment does not go as well as they expect.

Pitta types, being natural leaders, like authority and are impressed with important credentials. Yet the people who can really help us inwardly are not always those who are most prominent in social status. To find real help, Pitta types need to be more receptive or they can get trapped in their own judgments, which have caused their problems in the first place. They should not look to those who can impress or dominate them, but to those who can help them in a kind but firm manner, and who do not get drawn into their competitive dramas.

Pittas are highly intelligent and expect to be convinced of the validity of the treatments they are taking. They need to use their critical insight to understand the cause of their problems, which reside in their own behavior, not to struggle with others or with themselves. They must awaken their discrimination in order to take control of their own lives. To do this they have to learn the right use of intelligence and self-examination.

Fire-types must be approached with tact and diplomacy. They do not like to be given directions or told what to do. One must appeal to their native intelligence and logic, letting them see for themselves the truth of things. Opposing them encourages their basic aggression and will not help them learn. They like to work in friendship or in common alliance toward a particular goal. Cool, calm and pleasant circumstances mitigate their fiery nature. They need helpful friends and work well with a person or principles they respect.

Once Pitta types know what they need to do and understand the efforts they must make, they are usually the best of the three types in implementing behavioral changes. However, they can be excessive or fanatic and must be moderate in their actions so that they do not burn themselves out by attempting too much. They tend to be either for or against something and see things in black-and-white. They must learn to seek a balanced view and become considerate and diplomatic in their actions.

Kapha

Having the amorphous and docile nature of water, Kapha types need to be stimulated and sometimes shocked into changing themselves. They do not take hints. Nor will they do all the things to which they have agreed. Often they must be confronted or criticized in order to change bad habits. They must be approached with force, determination and consistency. Unless they are made acutely aware of a problem they may try to live with it.

It is not enough if one explains their problem to them and how to rectify it. They need an additional outside push, which may require regular repetition. A firm warning may be necessary to make them take heed of what they are doing. They must be made to see vividly the negative effects of their wrong lifestyles.

Water-types are slow to act and find it hard to implement things even after they accept them as necessary. They get bogged down in their own inertia and stagnation and find it difficult to start anything new. They are prone to addictions and to depression that prevents them from developing the proper initiative to improve themselves. They should not be comforted and consoled, though they may seek it. Their sentimentality about their condition is one of the factors that sustains it. Most of their problems arise from excess emotionality and can only be changed by a higher love or by detachment.

Kapha types are slow to respond and have difficulty discussing their problems. They need to open up slowly but require determination in order to do so. They must be coaxed out of their complacency. They may be bewildered by too much information. They respond better to prescriptions to make certain changes that are consistent and determined. They tend to return to their old habits even if they know they are bad, particularly if these are reinforced by the environment around them.

They need more frequent appointments with therapists and more constant interchange to stimulate them to get started. However, once started, which may take some time, they will usually continue well on their own accord. They must break their old deep-seated patterns and establish a new equilibrium before we can let them continue on their own. Once this is done, their lives can proceed smoothly on a peaceful basis. They can be as easily accustomed to a healthy flow in their lives as an unhealthy flow. The difficulty is in the transition.

Vata-Pitta

Vata-Pitta types have the volatility of air and fire combined. Fear and anger mix within them in an unpredictable way. If something does not make them afraid, it makes them mad. They are apt to be defensive and suspicious and find it difficult to trust anyone. They move from aggressive to defensive attitudes, from self-justification to criticizing others.

They require a great deal of tact and must strive to be patient with themselves. At times they may just be looking for someone upon whom they can unload their negativity. Often their energy reserves and immune system are not good (their Ojas tends to be low). For this reason, they may find it difficult to stand any criticism. They require much nurturing, patience and consideration (water). They need to create a lifestyle in which they take care of themselves, and in which others can help them to do so. They need a supportive environment and must allow other people to share their work.

Vata-Pitta types are usually highly intelligent, however, and once they feel calm and supported they can effectively implement a helpful line of treatment. However, their volatility can always erupt and must be guarded against. They must be consistent but gentle in their life-regimens and avoid excesses of all types. They benefit from a maternal (Kapha) force that grounds them.

Pitta-Kapha

Pitta-Kaphas have both energy (fire) and stability (water) and are generally the strongest physically of the different types. They have good resistance and are generally very healthy. They are strong and content in who they are and what they do. Psychologically, they are also strong and they are the least likely to seek out a therapist unless they have been unsuccessful in life.

Pitta-Kapha types lack adaptability and flexibility (air). They prefer to be dominating and controlling and tend to be conservative and possessive. This leads them to eventual suffering and frustration because most of life must remain beyond our power. They often break down later in life after they have failed in some major enterprise. In their case, such failures are often blessings in disguise and help them look within.

While they may be successful in the outer world, they may have difficulties in spiritual practices unless they learn to develop lightness, detachment and surrender. They require more activity, creativity and new challenges (more Prana). They need to learn to move on from what they have succeeded in and not get caught in power and control. Once settled in a line of treatment, they do well unless they get attached to their progress. For this reason it is best for them to have some variety in their treatment and not turn their therapy into a new form of achievement or acquisition.

Vata-Kapha

Vata-Kapha types lack energy, motivation, passion, and enthusiasm. They simply do not have the fire to get going in life, however much they may want to. They are often weak, passive, dependent, hypersensitive, and extremely yin. They will agree with what they are told but will lack the energy to put it into action. They are both emotionally and mentally (nervously) unstable, easily disturbed and frightened. They possess amorphous or chameleon personalities and will appear as you want them to be. Their judgment and discrimination tends to be poor and they easily get carried away by wrong associations or emotional influences.

On the positive side, Vata-Kapha types are sensitive, humble and adaptable. They can be highly artistic, imaginative or creative. They are considerate of others. They have no violence or ill-will toward anyone but blame themselves. They tend to be naive and need to be more realistic about other people and their motivations. They have to be careful not to let themselves be used or controlled. For this they need to be more assertive and challenge their fears.

They respond to warmth and firmness but it is hard for them to be consistent in their responses. They must learn to develop clarity, motivation and determination. They are most likely to develop dependency on their therapists and become addicted to their problems. However, once they turn their deep sensitivity in the right direction, they can contact inner sources of love and grace and themselves develop healing powers.

Vata-Pitta-Kapha Types

In some individuals, all three biological humors exist in relatively equal proportions. Treatment for them usually involves dealing with the biological humor currently out of balance. On a psychological level as well their condition can be changing. They need adaptability in their treatment and comprehensiveness of approach. Generally it is best to deal with any Vata problems they may have first, particularly through psychological therapies, because Vata is the most likely of the biological humors to cause problems. Pitta problems can be dealt with second, because these are the next problematical, and Kapha problems third because these are the least.

Balancing Therapy for the Mind

The Ayurvedic method of treatment is to relieve a negative condition by applying therapies of an opposite nature. If Vata (air) is too high, for example, its qualities of coldness, dryness, lightness and agitation will be elevated. This manifests in symptoms like cold extremities, dry skin, constipation, loss of body weight, or insomnia. Opposite therapies, like a rich nutritive diet, warm oil massage, rest and relaxation, are necessary to counter these.

The same principle holds true for the mind. A psychological imbalance is treated with opposite qualities to restore balance. This method for the mind is called Prati-paksha-Bhavana in Sanskrit.[50] It has been translated as "thinking thoughts of an opposite nature." However, its implications go beyond our surface thinking patterns. It means to "cultivate a balanced state of consciousness." For example, if our minds are disturbed by anger, we must cultivate peace. This requires not only thinking peaceful thoughts but taking in peaceful impressions, visualizing peace between ourselves and others, doing prayers for peace, and intentionally acting toward others, even our enemies, in a peaceful manner. It requires a complete lifestyle discipline.

Our consciousness is the result of the food, impressions, and associations to which we have become accustomed. It is reinforced by our actions and expressions. Whatever external force conditions us, we make it our own by expressing it. For example, if I am surrounded by anger as a child, I will likely become an angry person. When I act in an angry manner, then this anger, whose original impetus was external, becomes part of my own nature and automatic responses.

The influence of our daily lives creates a subtle imprint. It colors our consciousness just as a dye colors a cloth. This permeation of our consciousness by the subtle influences of our lives predisposes us to certain attitudes, which determine our mental happiness or unhappiness. The food, impressions and associations that we habituate ourselves have a permeating effect upon the mind. This permeating action goes deeper than our conscious thoughts. Most of it affects us on a subconscious level, as we note through how advertising manipulates us by appealing to instinctual responses like sex. To counter these deep-seated tendencies, an opposite type influence is required, an appeal to the subconscious but directed in a higher way toward healing and wholeness.

To change harmful mental conditions, we must cultivate an opposite way of consciousness, which means to create an opposite way of living. For example, if we are depressed we should eat vitalizing food. We should open ourselves up to the vital impressions of nature: the trees, flowers, and sunshine. We should associate with people who are creative and spiritual. We should not cultivate the thought that we are depressed. Rather we should cultivate the thought that we have energy, that we are not dependent upon anyone or anything else to make us happy. This requires understanding the part of our nature that is inherently free from psychological problems, our deeper Self.

According to Vedic thought, our original nature is good, beneficent and full. We are nothing but the Divine Self in incarnation. However, we obscure our original nature through contact with external conditioning factors. We take on a false or artificial nature, an ego identity that leads to sorrow. Whatever problem we have psychologically is not our true nature but a superimposition, a result of wrong conditioning; to look at it Ayurvedicly, it is just an expression of mental indigestion.

We often naturally try to counter our psychological problems with opposite influences, but in the wrong way, and therefore fail. For example, if we are depressed, we look for someone to cheer us up. If we cannot find such a person we get more depressed. Or we look for a stimulant. We drink coffee or alcohol, or take an anti-depressant. Such external stimulants breed dependency and leave us more depressed when they are not at our disposal. The method we are trying is correct, which is to counter our negative condition with an opposite positive energy, but our application is faulty. We are relying on substances that merely mask our condition but cannot resolve it. We are not ourselves creatively and consciously participating in the process. We must create a positive energy within our own mind and behavior to counter negative psychological conditions. We can benefit from positive external influences but should avoid those which breed addiction or dependency.

This cultivation of a balanced state of mind should not be confused with simple positive thinking. It is more than that. It requires not just thinking we are happy when we are sad, which may be only a fantasy, but also changing the conditions that make us unhappy, including our thoughts and our actions. We should not cover over thoughts of unhappiness with thoughts of happiness, but affirm the deeper happiness at the core of our being. For a balancing therapy to work, we must know how the qualities of things affect us. The following chapters examine the role of food, impressions, and associations so we can apply them to return to this original state of harmony that is inherent in our original nature.

11. The Cycle of Nutrition for the Mind: The Role of Impressions

How can we have a healthy mind? How can our consciousness, like the body, become strong, flexible, resilient and enduring? Just as there are rules for creating physical health, so there are rules for creating mental health. Most importantly, just as the body needs the right nutrition for health, so does the mind.

The mind is an organic entity, a part of Nature, and has its cycle of nutrition that involves taking in substances to build it up, like impressions, and releasing waste materials that can become toxins, like negative emotions. Food for the mind, like that for the body, creates the energy that allows it to work. Like the body, the mind has its proper exercise and expression, which requires the right food to sustain it.

Though most of us consider how we feed our bodies, we seldom consider how we feed our minds. We are often so caught up in our emotional impulses that we do not nourish our minds properly. As a result, our minds become distorted. Their natural urge toward light and knowledge becomes warped into seeking pleasure and self-aggrandizement. To change the mind, we must change what we feed it. Unless what we put into the mind changes, we cannot change what comes out of it. But what are the substances that feed the mind? Unless we know this we cannot go very far in treating the mind.

In this chapter we will examine in detail all the main factors of mental nutrition and mental digestion. Various methods will be provided to improve our mental nutrition and increase our capacity of mental digestion.

Physical — Food

The first level of nourishment for the mind comes through the food we take in, which provides the gross elements of earth, water, fire, air and ether. The essence of digested food serves to build up not only the brain and nerve tissue but also the subtle matter of the mind (note chapter on Diet and Herbs). The five gross elements build up the physical body directly and, indirectly, the mind. For example, the earth element in the food we take, like proteins, builds the heavy matter of the body, like the muscles, and helps ground and stabilize the mind through increasing the earth element within it.

Subtle — Impressions

The second level of nourishment for the mind comes through the impressions and experiences we take in through the senses. Through the senses we take in impressions from the external world: the colors, shapes, and sounds around us, which constitute the subtle elements. The five sensory potentials directly build up the outer mind (Manas) and indirectly the inner mind or deeper consciousness (Chitta). Sensory impressions color our thoughts and affect our feelings. The mind (Manas) itself brings in mental and emotional impressions that most strongly affect it.

Corresponding Gross and Subtle Elements

1) Earth   smell

2) Water   taste

3) Fire   sight

4) Air   touch

5) Ether   sound

6) Mind   mental and emotional impressions

Causal — Gunas

The third and deepest level of nutrition for the mind, which determines the nature of our deeper consciousness (Chitta), is through the three gunas of Sattva, Rajas and Tamas. The gross and subtle elements (food and impressions) affect our deeper consciousness according to their constituent gunas. Most importantly, we are affected by the gunas of the people we associate with at a heart level. After all, our relationships make the greatest impression upon us. This is why right relationship is so crucial in treating the mind. Our deeper consciousness is the level of the heart.

The gunas are the primal level of matter (Prakriti) and cannot be destroyed, but they can be transformed, which is what our food, impressions and associations affect. Sattvic food, impressions and associations activate the Sattvic qualities of consciousness like love, clarity and peace. Rajasic food, impressions and associations activate its Rajasic qualities like passion, criticalness and agitation. Tamasic food, impressions and associations activate the Tamasic qualities of insensitivity, ignorance and inertia. Chitta, our deeper consciousness, is the ultimate product of digestion of food, impressions and associations. To have a healthy consciousness requires that we consider all three levels of nutrition. Impressions and associations go together as the basic factors of our experience.

Mental Digestion

We must not only consider the nature of the food we take in but also our capacity to digest it. Even if we take good food, if our digestion is weak, it may turn into toxins. The mind, like the body, has its digestive power or digestive fire (Agni) which is intelligence (Buddhi).

The mind exists to provide experience and liberation for the soul. Experience that we have digested or understood brings freedom and allows for the expansion of awareness, just as food we have digested releases energy that allows us to work. Experience that we have not digested becomes a toxin and initiates various pathological changes in the mind, just as undigested food causes the disease process in the physical body. Just as well-digested food brings physical happiness and undigested food causes disease, so well-digested experience brings mental happiness, and poorly digested experience causes mental disorders.

The mind has its own pattern of digestion which resembles that of the physical body.

1. Outer Mind and Senses — Gathering of Impressions

The five senses bring in impressions, much like the hands and the mouth bring in food. These are gathered in the outer mind (Manas), which organizes them but does not have the power to digest them. The outer mind corresponds to the stomach in the physical body, which gathers and homogenizes food but cannot fully break it down or absorb it.

2. Intelligence — Digestion of Experience

Once the outer mind has gathered and homogenized our impressions, intelligence (Buddhi) works to digest them. Intelligence is the Agni or digestive fire for the mind and corresponds to the small intestine as a physical organ. Intelligence digests impressions and turns them into experiences. It turns present events into memories.

Proper mental digestion depends upon proper function of intelligence, through which we discern the truth of our experience from its outer names and forms. It enables us to take in the Sattva guna from our experiences and release their Rajasic and Tamasic components. Wrong mental digestion occurs when we are unable to break down the names and forms of our experience into truth energies. Then the undigested names and forms accumulate in the mind and block its perception. We mistake the appearance of things for their meaning or truth content. [51]

3. Consciousness — Absorption of Experience

Once intelligence has digested our impressions, they pass in the form of experience or memory into our deeper consciousness (Chitta), which they affect according to their qualities (gunas). Experience absorbed in the deeper consciousness becomes part of its fabric, just as the food digested becomes part of the tissue of the physical body. If our experience is not digested properly, it damages the substance of the mind, just as undigested food damages the tissues of the body. Experience that we have digested does not leave a mark or scar upon the mind in the form of memories, but allows us to function in life with peace and clarity.

Let us examine some examples of this process. If we see a beautiful sunset with an open heart this impression is easily digested and leaves an energy of light and peace in our deeper consciousness. If someone attacks or robs us, however, our mind gets disturbed. The experience is hard to digest, and leaves a residue of anger, frustration or fear. Our lives are filled with many such examples. Undigested experiences re-arise from our subconscious, influencing our current state of mind, until we understand and resolve them.

The Three States of Waking, Dream, and Deep Sleep

In the waking state we gather impressions through the outer mind (Manas) and senses. In the dream state we digest impressions through our inner intelligence (Buddhi) and these are reflected through our subtle senses in the form of various dreams. In deep sleep, the residue of our digested impressions, reduced to seed form, becomes part of our deeper consciousness (Chitta).

Our dreams show the process of mental digestion. Good dreams reflect good mental digestion. Bad dreams show poor mental digestion.[52] Similarly, good deep sleep reflects a well-developed body of consciousness. Inability to sustain deep sleep shows a poorly developed body of consciousness.

Detoxification for the Mind

Detoxification is just as necessary for the mind as it is for the body. Yet for detoxification to begin we must first stop taking toxins into ourselves. For mental well-being, there must be first a prevention of wrong impressions and experiences from entering into our consciousness, just as for physical well-being we must avoid wrong food.

Second, there must be a strong intelligence to digest impressions properly. We must strive to avoid negative experiences as much as possible. When we cannot do this, we must have enough intelligence to digest even disturbing impressions, which are not always avoidable. Eliminating toxins from the consciousness involves stopping their intake, which requires control of the mind and senses. Then it requires directing the light of intelligence within to burn up the wrong experiences we have already absorbed.

Just as fasting from food helps detoxify the body, so fasting from impressions detoxifies the mind. Once the intake of impressions ceases, consciousness, whose nature is space, will naturally empty itself out. Its contents will come up to the level of the intelligence which can then digest them properly. This requires deep thinking, inquiry and meditation. When the outer mind and senses are calm and quiet, our inner thoughts arise. Deep-seated habits and memories float to the surface. If we learn to observe and understand them, we can let them go, but this requires that we are willing to be free from them.

Physical Level of Detoxification — Pure Diet

Toxic accumulations of the gross elements, mainly earth and water, are eliminated from the physical body through ordinary elimination channels of excretion, urination and sweating. Special Ayurvedic detoxification measures help us release excesses of the three Doshas along with these waste materials.[53] Fasting is another important measure, which allows the body to burn up toxins. Special herbs can help as well.

Subtle Level of Detoxification — Pranayama

Negative impressions (the subtle elements) are eliminated mainly through Pranayama or yogic breathing exercises, which create a special type of sweating that releases excess subtle water and earth elements (taste and odor). Ordinary sweating therapies help in this process, including use of sweat lodges, steam baths, saunas and diaphoretic (sweat-inducing) herbs. Sweating therapy is part of Ayurvedic Pancha Karma therapy, which aids in the purification of the subtle as well as the gross body. Fasting from impressions (Pratyahara) is another helpful method, which, like fasting from food, allows undigested and toxic impressions to be released. Crying, a sincere flow of tears reflecting a real change of heart, is another way that the mind can be purified of negative emotions.

Causal Level of Detoxification — Mantra

The gunas are the core level of matter and are indestructible. There is no release of the gunas from consciousness (Chitta) but they can be transformed. Toxic accumulations of the gunas (excess Rajas and Tamas) can be changed into Sattva. This occurs through mantra or sound therapy. Sattvic mantras like OM help change the Rajasic and Tamasic patterns in our deeper consciousness and make it Sattvic. They change the fabric of the Chitta and make it receptive to higher influences.

Cultivating the Field of Consciousness

Consciousness (Chitta) is a field and like the earth has a feminine and creative quality. What we put into it, in terms of our life-experience, is how we cultivate this field. According to how we cultivate it, so things will grow within it. If our field of consciousness is cultivated with good food and impressions, then bad habits and impulses will not have a favorable environment in which to take root. If we take in bad food and impressions, then even good thoughts and impulses will have no favorable ground on which to grow.

We can again draw a physical comparison. If we build up our bodily tissues with wrong food, the tissues themselves will be damaged or deficient. Once the structure of the body is damaged, it becomes difficult to maintain health. Similarly, consciousness has its substance that is created through time. If it is wrongly developed, like a wrongly grown tree, it can require much time and effort to fix, if it can be fixed at all.

Consciousness is also like a deep well. What we take in through the senses and mind are like the things that we throw into the well. We do not see the effects of what we take in because the well is so deep. Yet whatever we throw into the well of consciousness grows according to its nature and will eventually impel us to act. Nothing that we put into our consciousness remains static or has no effect. Consciousness is fertile and creative. Whatever we deposit in it has its progeny, which we will have to deal with for good or ill.

We must be very careful in how we feed our minds. The results will manifest over time, after which it may be too late to reverse if these are negative. We must constantly guard our consciousness and what we put into it. We must treat it like a delicate flower that requires proper soil and nutrients. We must protect it from wrong influences and associations as if it were a child. This requires a clear intelligence and a consistent life regimen in harmony with our nature.

Factors of Mental Nutrition

For treating disease, physical or mental, we must consider the following factors of nutrition: 1) Proper food and drink; 2) Proper air and right breathing; and 3) Proper impressions. Proper food, drink and air nourishes the physical body and the Pranas. Proper impressions nourish the outer mind and senses. Our impressions serve as vehicles for the feelings, emotions, beliefs, values and attitudes that nourish our intelligence and deeper consciousness.

For properly nourishing the mind, Ayurveda employs certain techniques involving positive impressions, emotions, thoughts, beliefs, and attitudes. The physical side of mental nutrition or food is dealt with in the chapter on diet and herbs. The use of the breath is examined in the chapter on Yoga relative to Pranayama. In the remainder of this chapter we will examine internal factors that affect the mind, primarily various types of impressions.

Sensory Impressions

The senses are our main gates to the external world, through which we take in not only sensory but mental and emotional influences. The proper and balanced use of the senses makes us healthy and happy. The improper, excessive or deficient use of the senses makes us unhealthy and disturbed. Our senses are constantly feeding us with impressions, which determine who we are and what will we become.[54]

We are constantly bringing in sensory impressions of all types that must affect us in their different ways. We spend much of our time taking in special sensory impressions through various forms of recreation and entertainment. However, most of the time we are so engrossed in the world of the senses, like watching a movie, that we fail to step back and examine what is happening to us through our sensory interactions.

The intake of impressions is a subtle form of eating in which certain nutrients are taken in from external objects. This we can easily observe by seeing how our daily impressions reverberate in our minds when we sleep through the kinds of dreams that they create. For example, if we have been caught in hectic traffic in a noisy and polluted part of a large city, our minds will also feel noisy and polluted. On the other hand, positive impressions, like those gathered during a hike or walk in the woods, will make the mind feel expansive and peaceful.

However, many people today, including those in the medical field, do not accept that sensory impressions influence the mind. This debate is most noticeable in the issue of television violence, which many people claim does not make those who watch it more violent. To Ayurveda, this is like saying the food we eat does not affect our health. Ayurveda states that the impressions we take in affect our behavior directly. Watching television violence may not make us overtly violent, but it does not make us non-violent. And it certainly makes us dull and dependent upon external stimulation of a distorted nature.

The mind is very sensitive to impressions. Our impressions feed our life-force and motivate our actions. Disturbed impressions cause disturbed expressions. Peaceful impressions cause peaceful expressions. Only if we have a great deal of inner awareness can we effectively ward off the negative impressions that we all must contact to some degree.

Impressions are taken in by the outer mind based upon its receptivity to them. They are judged or digested by the intelligence and their residue is deposited in the feeling nature or consciousness. There, any residue of wrong impressions become inherent as an obstruction in the mental field, which gives rise to various wrong perceptions and actions. We do not automatically absorb sensory influences. We can discriminate them away through the proper function of intelligence. This requires discerning their truth and not getting caught in their glamour.

There is a whole science of impressions. Just as the food we eat can be examined through our digestion and elimination, the effects of impressions can be observed in various ways. Many mental disorders arise from the intake of wrong impressions and can be cured through the intake of right impressions. As it is easier to change our impressions than to alter our thoughts and emotions, impressions allow us perhaps the simplest way to change the entire mental field.

Signs of Proper Intake of Impressions

acuity of sensory functioning
control of the imagination
deep sleep with few or with spiritual dreams
lack of need for entertainment
clear perception, capacity for creative expression
mental lightness, peace and luminosity

Signs of Improper Intake of Impressions

improper functioning of the senses
disturbed imagination
disturbed sleep, frequent or agitated dreams
craving for violent or disturbed entertainment
unclear perception, lack of creativity
mental heaviness, disturbance and darkness

Positive and Negative Impressions

The main source of positive impressions is Mother Nature herself — the impressions gained from the sky, mountains, forests, gardens, rivers and ocean. Is there anyone who is not elevated by being in beautiful natural surroundings? A great portion of our modern psychological unrest is simply due to alienation from Nature that deprives us of the impressions natural to our mental well-being. Instead of taking in positive natural impressions, we fill the mind with artificial sensations from our artificial world. Just like junk food affects the body, such "junk impressions" must distort the mind.

We can create our own positive impressions. Much of what is called good art is an attempt to create a higher level of impressions that reflect our inner being. Religion aims at this through ritual, mantra or visualization.

Any impression apart from nature, genuine art or spirituality must have some negative consequences. The main source of negative impressions today is through the mass media, though not all mass media impressions are bad. Impressions gained in artificial environments like roads or cities are also disturbing. Those gained in personal conflicts or other problems with people can also be very negative.

Negative impressions, like junk food, become addicting. As junk food has little real nutritional content or natural taste, it must be made palatable by adding large amounts of salt, sugar or spices. As it has no real nutritional content, we are compelled to take more of it, trying to gain some nourishment from it. The spice for negative impressions is sex and violence. Because there is no real life in mass media impressions, we must give them the illusion of life by portraying the most dramatic events in life.

We can take in positive impressions in two ways: first in terms of the immediate home environment, second in terms of the general environment, which includes the workplace, society and the world of nature. To nourish the mind, we must have beauty and harmony in our home environment. We must have a place of peace and happiness. To bring this about, it may be necessary to create a sacred or healing space in the house. There are various ways to do this. Generally a room should be set aside for spiritual and creative activity. An altar can be set up with pictures of deities or gurus, sacred objects like statues, gems or crystals, or harmonious shapes, colors or geometrical designs. Incense, flowers, fragrances, bells or music can be used. Some prayer, meditation or relaxation should be done daily at this place.

Ideally our house should be a temple, but at least one portion of it should be kept as a place of healing and meditation where we can go to be renewed. We should resort to such a healing room whenever our physical or mental energy is drained. In severe cases, a patient may have to stay in such a healing room for extended periods.

In terms of our external environment, we must reestablish our communion with nature. We should spend a certain amount of time regularly in communion with nature. We can go hiking, camping or merely work in the garden. We must draw into our lives the energy of the sky, mountains, plains and waters. We must link up with the cosmic life-force that alone has the power to heal our individual life-force. Our individual life-force cannot heal itself if it becomes a closed system, apart from Nature.

We must bring higher impressions into our workplace. Perhaps a small portion of it can be made into an altar or at least a garden. We must bring higher impressions into

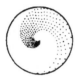

our social interaction. This can be done by going to spiritual places like temples, doing chants, rituals or meditations in a group.

Impressions to Reduce the Three Doshas

The following pages provide an outline of impressions to reduce the Doshas. These are explained in detail in the appropriate chapters on diet, herbs, aromas, color therapy, mantra, Yoga and meditation.

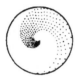

Vata-reducing Impressions

Nature: sitting or walking quietly and peacefully by a garden, forest, river, lake or ocean, particularly where it is warm and bright

Sensory:
1. sound — calming music and chanting, classical music, chanting, peaceful silence
2. touch — gentle and warming touch or massage, using warm oils like sesame or almond
3. sight — bright and calming colors like combinations of gold, orange, blue, green, white
4. taste — rich and nourishing food abounding in sweet, salty and sour tastes, with moderate use of spices
5. smell — sweet, warm, calming and clearing fragrances like jasmine, rose, sandalwood, eucalyptus

Activity: gentle exercise, Hatha Yoga (particularly seated and inverted postures), Tai Chi, swimming, hot tubs (but do not stay in too long), relaxation, more sleep

Emotional: cultivating peace, contentment, fearlessness and patience; releasing fear and anxiety, having the support of good friends and family with regular social interaction

Mental: anti-Vata mantras like Ram, Hrim or Shrim, concentration exercises, strengthening memory

Spiritual: meditation on strong, benefic, happy or peaceful deities like Rama and Krishna, or protective forms of the Divine Mother (like Durga or Tara) or Divine Father, prayers for peace and protection, developing discrimination and insight

Pitta-reducing impressions

Nature: sitting or walking by flowers, river, lake or ocean, particularly when it is cool; walking at night, gazing at the night sky, moon and stars

Sensory:
1. Sound — cooling and soft music like the sound of flutes, sound of water
2. Touch — cooling, soft and moderate touch and massage with cooling oils like coconut or sunflower

3. Sight — cool colors like white, blue and green
4. Taste — food that is neither too heavy nor too light, abounding in sweet, bitter and astringent tastes, with few spices except those that are cooling like coriander, turmeric and fennel
5. Smell — cool and sweet fragrances like rose, sandalwood, vetivert, champak, gardenia or jasmine

Activity: moderate exercise, walking, swimming, cooling Asanas like shoulder stand

Emotional: cultivating friendship, kindness and courtesy, promoting peace, forgiveness, compassion and devotion; releasing anger, resentment, conflict and hatred

Mental: anti-Pitta mantras like Shrim, Sham or Ma, practicing non-judgment and acceptance, listening to other people's points of view

Spiritual: meditation on benefic and peaceful deities like Shiva (in his peaceful form), Vishnu or benefic forms of the Divine Mother (like Lakshmi); prayers for universal peace, cultivating surrender and receptivity

Kapha-reducing impressions

Nature: vigorous hiking or walking in dry or desert regions, high mountains, or on sunny and windy days in open areas

Sensory:
1. Sound — stimulating music, strong and energizing sounds, singing
2. Touch — strong, deep body massage with dry powders or stimulating oils like mustard
3. Sight — bright and stimulating colors like yellow, orange, gold and red
4. Taste — light diet emphasizing pungent, bitter and astringent tastes with liberal use of spices, occasional fasting
5. Smell — light, warm, stimulating and penetrating fragrances like musk, cedar, myrrh, camphor and eucalyptus

Activity: strong aerobic exercise, jogging, sunbathing, wind-bathing, saunas, reducing sleep

Emotional: cultivating detachment, service to others and selfless love; releasing greed, attachment, and clinging

Mental: anti-Kapha mantras like Aim, Krim or Hum, cultivating wakefulness, mental exercises and games (like chess), breaking with the past and with tradition

Spiritual: meditation on active or wrathful Deities, including strong forms of the Divine Mother (like Kali) or of the Divine Father (like Rudra), meditation on the Void or on the inner light

12. Outer Treatment Modalities: Diet, Herbs, Massage and Pancha Karma

Treating the mind is unlikely to be successful if we do not also consider the condition of the body. In this chapter we will examine the physical treatment methods of Ayurveda and how they can be used relative to the mind. These begin with the most basic factors, which are diet, herbs and massage. Because they are explained in detail in regular Ayurveda books, we will only examine them generally.

Diet

The food that we eat affects not only our body but our entire state of mind. As is the quality of our food, so becomes the quality of our consciousness. Similarly, unless we change our diet, we are unlikely to be able to change our consciousness. We can all easily observe how different foods affect us. Food that is heavy, like steak, makes the mind heavy and can cause irritability, dullness and depression. Food that is light, like fruit or salads, makes the mind light, and in excess causes lightheadedness and insomnia. Food that is balanced and full of the life-force, like whole grains and cooked vegetables, improves sensory function and promotes mental harmony and clarity. If we want to calm our emotions or raise our state of consciousness, we cannot ignore the food we eat or our dietary habits.

Diet is one of the most important therapies in Ayurveda. In fact, Ayurvedic treatment begins with the proper
diet. The physical body, after all, is made up of food which
builds the tissues. While diet is not central to treating
psychological conditions, it cannot be ignored. An
Ayurvedic diet can be a very helpful factor for treating the
mind. This section does not aim at outlining a complete
Ayurvedic dietary therapy. That can be gained from other
books on Ayurveda.[55] Here we will deal primarily with the
mental and emotional effects of food.

Food provides three levels of nutrition: 1) Physical
(outer level) — five elements; 2) Mental (inner level) —
sensory and mental impressions; and 3) Spiritual (core
level) — three gunas.

Food itself is a physical substance composed of the five
elements of earth, water, fire, air and ether. It provides the
first or physical level of nutrition directly, the other two
indirectly. The second and third levels of nutrition occur
on the levels of the mind (Manas) and consciousness (Chitta) respectively. This was discussed in the chapters relating
to sensory therapies and the functions of the mind.

However, because food affects the other levels of our
nature through a physical medium, it takes its influence
deep into the unconscious. Food nourishes the vital force
that sustains autonomic and instinctual reflexes. Through
the vital force, the effects of food can reach the emotional
urges embedded in our deeper consciousness. Through the
vital-force, the food drives us to particular activities.
according to its nature. For example, if we eat a lot of
meat, which is permeated with the influence of harm to
other creatures, this will promote aggressive and perhaps
violent actions on our part.

During the process of eating, our life-force and mind

open up and are exposed to environmental influences. Our Prana becomes exposed. While eating we become vulnerable to impressions and feelings from the world around us. We are strongly influenced by people while eating with them, particularly in social circumstances, like in a restaurant. We are not only what we eat but whom we eat with, as well as where we eat.

The impulses of the unconscious are the hardest part of awareness to change and the source of the hidden fears and desires that most disturb us. Therefore we should not underestimate the power of food to affect either our thoughts or our behavior. Control of diet aids in the control of the subconscious and the release of its contents. As psychological problems are rooted in the unconscious, diet should not be overlooked in treating them.

Most psychological problems reflect our dietary habits, either in what or how we eat. They cause us to eat wrong food or to eat in a wrong or irregular manner. All imbalances of the mind disturb the digestive system through the nervous system. Correcting diet helps clear out the unconscious habits that sustain our mental unrest.

Levels of Nutrition Through Food

Food provides nourishment through all the five elements, predominantly earth. The six tastes of food help build up the respective elements in the body and mind (see table below).

Element	In	Nourishes
Earth	Solid food	Internal organs, muscles, skin, bones and other earth predominant tissues
Water	Liquid food	Mucous membranes, secretions, plasma, fat, And drink nerve, reproductive and other liquid predominant tissues
Fire	Heat, sunlight and fire element in food	Blood, digestive fire, and fire predominant enzymes and digestive juices
Air	Breath and the air element in food	Vitalizes nervous system, promotes discharge of impulses and secretions
Ether	Space in breath and in food	Clears and nourishes mind and senses

Along with the food we eat, we take in various sensory impressions, the most evident being the taste of the food, although smell, texture, and sight also come into play. Additional subtle impressions come in through how the food is grown and prepared, as well as the atmosphere and state of mind in which it is eaten. This is part of the second or mental level of nutrition.

Food, like all things in the universe, consists of the three cosmic qualities of Sattva (balance), Rajas (agitation) and Tamas (resistance). These are reflected in both the elements and impressions gained through the food. These constitute the third or core level of nutrition, which Ayurveda emphasizes through a Sattvic diet.

Sattvic Diet

Ayurveda emphasizes a Sattvic diet for healthful living, particularly for keeping our minds happy and at peace.

Sattvic diet was originally devised for the practice of Yoga and the development of higher consciousness. It aids in the treatment of mental disorders because it helps restore harmony and balance (Sattva) to the mind.

The prime factor in a Sattvic diet is vegetarian food. If one follows a vegetarian diet, one goes a long way toward a wholesome diet for the mind. This means avoiding meat and fish, and all other foods caused by harming animals.[56] Red meat is the worst in this regard, particularly beef.

Yet being a vegetarian does not require following a strict raw food diet, living only on salads and fresh fruit. The cerebrospinal fluid has an oily nature and needs certain rich foods to sustain it. Nutritive vegetarian foods like whole grains, seeds, nuts, and dairy products help build the brain tissue and develop Ojas. Raw foods, like salads and greens, detoxify the body and increase Prana, but are not adequate to sustain our energy over long periods of time, particularly if we do physical work or movement.

Sattvic diet means not only vegetarian food, but food rich in Prana (life-force) like organic fresh fruit and vegetables. It requires avoiding canned and processed food, and foods prepared with chemical fertilizers or sprays. It also means properly cooked fresh food. Even if we cook food, we should make sure that it is fresh to begin with, eaten at the same meal and not overcooked.

It takes time for the effects of dietary changes to manifest on the mind. Changing our diet may not impact our psychology overnight, but in a period of months can affect it significantly. A number of psychological disorders can be cured, or at least alleviated, by following a Sattvic diet as outlined in the appendix. While it may not be possible to follow a strictly Sattvic diet, we should at least orient our food habits in that direction. For psychological imbalances, we should consider diet more seriously.

Sattvic Diet and the Six Tastes

Ayurveda recognizes six tastes, each of which is composed of two of the five elements:

Sweet ....earth and water

Salty ....water and fire

Sour ....earth and fire

Pungent ....fire and air

Bitter ....air and ether

Astringent..................earth and air

Sweet is the primary Sattvic taste because it is nurturing and harmonizing, reflecting the energy of love. Pungent, sour and salty tastes are Rajasic (stimulant-irritant) because they activate the senses and make the mind extroverted. Bitter and astringent tastes are Tamasic in the long term because their effect is to deplete the vital fluids.

However, we need all six tastes to various degrees. The right balance of tastes itself is Sattvic. This consists of food that is pleasant, but not overly sweet, in taste like grains, fruit and sweet vegetables, along with moderate use of spices, salt and condiments, and taking only bitter and astringent articles for necessary detoxification. Sattvic diet is mild and even in qualities, not going to any extreme of taste.

Pungent taste irritates the nerves by its stimulating and dispersing property. Sour and salty tastes aggravate the emotions through heating the blood. Bitter and astringent tastes can make us ungrounded and dry out the nervous system. However, a number of sweet spices, like ginger, cinnamon and cardamom, are Sattvic and help clear the mind and harmonize emotions. Some special bitter herbs, like gotu kola, are Sattvic. Bitter taste helps open the mind because it is composed of the same basic elements of air and ether.

Too much of any taste becomes Tamasic or dulling. This is particularly true of sweet taste, which is heavy in nature. We have all experienced the dulling effect of eating too many sweets. Complex carbohydrates are better for the mind than raw sugars. Pure sugars overstimulate the pancreas. They require the pancreas to work hard to keep blood sugar levels down when they enter the blood and, when they leave the blood, make it work hard to keep the blood sugar level up. This can cause mood swings and emotional imbalances. Because sweet taste is Sattvic or love-promoting, we indulge in it in order to compensate for lack of love in our lives.

Excessive eating is Tamasic, while light eating is Sattvic, though light eating can be Rajasic if food intake is not adequate to ground the mind. Overweight is a Tamasic state, causing dullness and heaviness in the mind, while underweight is Rajasic, promoting hypersensitivity and hyperactivity.

Rajasic and Tamasic Diets

Rajasic and Tamasic foods disturb or dull the mind and produce unrest and disease. We should understand them in order to avoid them. Rajasic food is excessively spicy, salty and sour: like chilies, garlic, onions, wines, pickles, excess salt, mayonnaise, sour cream, and vinegar. Food too hot in temperature is Rajasic. Rajasic food is usually taken with stimulating (Rajasic) beverages like coffee or alcohol. It may be eaten in Rajasic circumstances, as when we are hurried, disturbed or agitated.

Tamasic food is stale, old, recooked, rancid, artificial, overly fried, greasy or heavy. It includes all "dead" food, meat and fish, particularly pork, animal fats and animal organ parts. Canned and artificial foods tend to be Tamasic. Excess intake of fats, oils, sugars and pastries is Tamasic. White sugar and white flour have a long-term Tamasic or clogging effect (though short term white sugar is Rajasic). Food that is too cold is also Tamasic and weakens the digestive fire.

Rajasic foods cause hyperactivity and irritability, increase toxins in the blood, and promote hypertension. They disturb the senses and cause the emotions to fluctuate. Tamasic foods cause hypoactivity, lethargy, apathy, excess sleep, accumulate phlegm and waste materials. They dull the senses and keep the emotions heavy and resistant.

Sattvic Diet with Diets for the Three Humors

Sattvic diet can be modified for best effect according to the three biological humors of Vata, Pitta and Kapha. One should follow the diet for one's constitutional type, emphasizing those articles which are Sattvic and avoiding those which are Rajasic or Tamasic.[57] By combining a diet for increasing Sattva along with one for reducing one's biological humor, diet becomes a powerful tool for improving health. For specific psychological problems, more specialized diets may be prescribed. For specific information on Sattvic food types, note the appendix.

Herbs

Herbs are Mother Nature's primary medicine and carry her healing energies to keep our system in balance. Ayurveda is primarily an herbal medicine. Ayurvedic books explain herbal qualities and energetics in detail.[58] Here we will focus on how herbs can be used in a simple way relative to the mind. Herbs affect the mind more directly than food, though they are milder and safer in action than chemical drugs. They can be very important tools for healing the mind. While all herbs have some effect on the mind, certain herbs are nervines and possess a special action on the brain and nervous system.

Herbs work over a period of time, though shorter than that of food. Up to one month may be necessary for the effect of mild herbs to manifest, particularly those used for their nutritive effect. The exception is strong stimulant herbs (like cayenne or ma huang) which have an immediate effect.

Herbs in Ayurvedic Psychology

Ayurveda's integral psychology stresses first of all appropriate diet. On top of this, special herbs are helpful if not indispensable. Diet has a general role and provides the foundation on which herbs can work. Without the proper diet, even the best herbs will be limited in what they can do. Herbs are used for fine tuning diet and for shorter, but stronger therapeutic actions.[59] To understand the Ayurvedic view, it is necessary to understand the effects of the six tastes on the mind.[60]

The Six Tastes and the Mind

Bitter Taste

Bitter taste is composed of air and ether elements, which are the same elements as predominate in the mind. Bitter herbs open the mind, make consciousness more sensitive, and increase its functional capacity. They have a cooling, calming, detaching and expanding effect on the mind.

Those suffering from mental dullness, heaviness, heat and toxicity should use more of the bitter taste. However, bitter taste should not be used by those suffering from hyperactivity, nervous exhaustion, debility or ungrounded- edness. It is more for short term usage or in small dosages. Typical Bitter Nervines include betony, chamomile, gotu kola, hops, manduka parni, passion flower, and skullcap.

Pungent Taste

Pungent or spicy taste is composed of fire and air ele- ments and activates these in the mind. As the most fiery of the tastes, pungent is best for increasing Tejas and intelli- gence. Pungent herbs stimulate the mind and promote cir- culation in the brain. They help develop clarity, perception and reasoning ability.

Pungent herbs are good for those suffering from men- tal dullness, depression, congestion, and lack of motiva- tion. They should generally be avoided by those suffering from anger, insomnia, restlessness, or hyperactivity. They often work better in combination with sweet tonics, which ground and stabilize their effects.

Most pungent herbs serve as nervine stimulants. Spicy herbs open the mind and senses, clear the head and sinus- es, relieve headache, muscle spasms and nerve pain. Some are more specifically nervine than others, particularly those that help clear the sinuses. Typical herbs of this type include basil, bayberry, calamus, camphor, cardamom, eucalyptus, hyssop, peppermint, pippali, rosemary, saffron, sage, spearmint, thyme, and wintergreen.

Though most pungent (spicy) herbs are stimulating, a few are calming or sedative in nature. These are often strong and earthy in taste. They are particularly good for Vata. Such herbs are asafetida, garlic, jatamansi, nutmeg, valerian, and lady's slipper.

Classified within pungent taste are certain strong nervine stimulants owing to the special alkaloids they contain. These herbs help us stay awake and focused, but can also irritate the nerves. They are useful in a limited way in conditions of depression or dullness, but can aggravate insomnia, restlessness and anxiety, or increase nervous debility. Herbs in this category are coffee, damiana, ephedra, ma huang, tea, and yohimbe.

Sweet Taste

Sweet taste is composed of earth and water elements. It is used for grounding, calming and nutritive purposes for the mind and nerves, and can have rejuvenative effects. Such herbs are usually not strongly sweet in taste but only mildly so. Those suffering from congestion or depression should avoid sweet tonic nervines because these slow and consolidate our energy. The most important tonic nervines are ashwagandha, bala, vidari, gokshura, licorice, lotus seeds, sesame seeds, shatavari, and zizyphus seeds.

Salty Taste

Salty taste is composed of water and fire elements. This gives it sedative and grounding properties. It is not a common herb taste but occurs in seaweeds and sea shells. It is mainly used for conditions of nervous debility or hyperactivity, which are primarily Vata conditions. Ayurveda contains special preparations of various sea shells and coral. Calmative Nervine Salts and minerals include black salt, conch shell powder (shankha bhasma), kelp, oyster shell powder (mukti bhasma), pearl powder (moti bhasma), red coral powder (praval bhasma), and rock salt.

Astringent Taste

Astringent taste is composed of earth and air. It is little used for nervine purposes but can help heal nerve tissue and stop spasms. There are a few special nervines that help calm and heal the mind. Such astringent nervines are bayberry, frankincense, haritaki, nutmeg, myrrh, and guggul.

Sour Taste

Sour taste is composed of earth and fire. It is not much used for nervine purposes but is a mild stimulant and can help counter depression and dizziness. Sour substances like vinegar and alcohol help extract the alkaloids in some herbs and become the base of herbal wines and tinctures. Among sour nervines are amalaki, lime, tamarind, and wine.

Cleansing and Tonic Nervines

Herbs work as nutritive and cleansing agents on two primary levels. Nutritive agents are tonics that build up the tissues. These herbs contain mainly earth and water elements, like food, but of a subtler or predigested type. Cleansing agents are detoxifiers that facilitate natural cleansing processes, like sweating or urination. These herbs usually predominate in fire, air and ether elements. The following are the main cleansing actions herbs can have on the nervous system.

Expectorants and Decongestants: These herbs clear mucous (Kapha) from the head, which obstructs the functioning of the brain and senses, help open the channels of the nerves and sinuses and relieve pain. Such are bayberry, calamus, camphor, cinnamon, eucalyptus, ginger, peppermint, pippali, and wintergreen.

Alternatives and Antipyretics: These promote blood circulation, reduce heat and toxins from the brain. Such herbs may also promote urination, which aids in cleansing the nervous system through the blood. Typical herbs of this type include gotu kola, manduka parni, passion flower, sandalwood, skullcap, guggul, and myrrh.

Sedatives: These possess specific anti-pain properties and counter high Vata (air) conditions of insomnia, anxiety, fear and pain. Typical of such herbs are asafetida, garlic, jatamansi, lady's slipper, shankha pushpi, and valerian.

Tonic and rejuvenative agents strengthen our internal organs, tissues, systems and energies. Those that strengthen the body as a whole or the vital force improve the mind indirectly. Some are specifically tonics for the mind. Below are some of the main tonic herbs on different levels.

Tonics for the Biological Humors

Vata: amalaki, ashwagandha, bala, garlic, licorice, shatavari, vidari

Pitta: amalaki, aloe gel, bala, gotu kola, red coral, licorice, lotus seeds, shatavari

Kapha: aloe gel, ashwagandha, elecampane, garlic, guggul, myrrh, pippali, shilajit

Rejuvenatives for the Mind[61]: calamus, gotu kola, manduka parni, shankha pushpi

Taking Herbs

Herbs can be used to treat mild complaints and as general tonics for the mind. For this, their dosage should be about one gram of the powder or one teaspoon of the cut and sifted herb per cup of water, taken two or three times a day. High dosages of herbs or powerful herbs should be given by a practitioner. Herbs vary their action according to the medium (anupana) with which they are taken. Below we list the most important and commonly used of these mediums.

Ghee: Ghee is clarified butter. It is made by cooking butter (preferably raw and unsalted) over a low flame until all the milk fats settle to the bottom and the above liquid is clear. Ghee is an excellent vehicle with which to take nervine herbs. Ghee feeds the nerve tissue and guides the effects of herbs into it. Ghee is taken with tonic herbs to improve their nutritive properties and with bitter herbs for strengthening their cooling effects.

Honey: Honey has decongestant, expectorant and nutritive properties. It helps clear the head, mind and senses. It is a good vehicle to take with pungent or spicy nervines like bayberry, calamus, ginger or pippali.

Milk: Taking an herb in a milk decoction increases both its tonic and calmative properties. A quarter-teaspoon of nutmeg taken in a cup of warm milk, along with a little ghee, is a mild sedative-relaxant. A teaspoon of ashwagandha with a little nutmeg in a milk decoction is a good nervine tonic. Gotu kola prepared in milk is a mild herbal tonic. However, we should try to get good quality milk, raw if possible.

Tinctures

Tinctured herbs, owing to the properties of alcohol which are subtle and penetrating, have a more direct activity on the brain. The alcohol increases their anti-Kapha effects. Usually a mixture of half pure alcohol and half distilled water is used. Alcohol extracts only the fire, air and ether elements of which it is composed. It is best for stimulant and detoxifying actions, not for tonic actions. It can be boiled away for those wishing to avoid the alcohol.

Herbs and the Nose (Nasya)

One of the best ways to bring the effects of herbs into the brain and nervous system is to apply them through the nose. There are several ways to do this:

1) Aroma therapy and incense (discussed in a separate chapter)

2) Application of oils to the nose:

Sesame oil can be put into the nose for its calming and nurturing action. Ghee is especially good for soothing the nerves and for countering allergies. Coconut can be used in a similar manner. Apply a few drops of these oils with an eye dropper while the head is tilted. Or put some oil on the tip of your little finger and apply gently inside the nose.

3) Snuff of the powders of various herbs:

Snuff of calamus powder is one of the best ways to open the head and sinuses, stimulate blood flow to the brain, and bring great acuity to the voice and the senses.

Put some of the powdered herb on the outside of the index finger and inhale, closing the opposite nostril with a finger of the other hand.

Oil Massage

Oil massage (Abhyanga) is an important Ayurvedic therapy not only for physical but for psychological conditions. Oil massage is calming to the mind, nurturing to the heart, and strengthening to the bones and nerves. We should all get oil massage on a regular basis as part of a healthy life regimen, as well as using them to treat various diseases.

Oils should be applied warm. They should be left on for some time (at least fifteen minutes) for proper absorption. Afterwards one can take a shower or steam bath to remove the excess oil. To make this easier, apply a powder like calamus to absorb the excess oil and then rub off the powder.

Sesame Oil: Sesame oil is specific for lowering high Vata and increasing Ojas. It is very grounding and nurturing to the mind. Anti-Vata herbs like ashwagandha, calamus, nirgundi, fennel or ginger can be cooked in it to give it more strength.

Sesame oil can be applied to the head, hair, back or feet for calmative purposes, particularly in the evening. The oil should be left on for at least fifteen minutes, after which it can be washed off during a warm shower. For all people suffering from pain and anxiety, regular sesame oil massage is a must.

Coconut Oil: Coconut oil is specific for lowering high Pitta. It is cooling and calming to the mind, nerves and skin. Anti-Pitta herbs, particularly Brahmi (Gotu Kola) do well prepared in this oil. Coconut oil can be applied to the head, hair and sensory openings (like the ear drums and nostrils), as well as used as a general massage oil.

Mustard Oil: Mustard oil is specific for lowering high Kapha. It is warming, stimulating and improves circulation. It helps clear the channels of the lungs and head and is good for mental dullness and depression. It can be used as a general massage oil or massaged to cover regions, like the lungs.

Pancha Karma

Pancha Karma is the main Ayurvedic method of physical purification. Owing to the subtle nature of its processes, it penetrates deep into the nervous system. It is useful for psychological problems caused by excesses of the three doshas. Yet it can also be helpful for psychological problems caused by internal factors, emotions and karma. It consists of five main purification practices:

1) Therapeutic emesis for removing excess Kapha — good for dealing with depression, grief and attachment;

2) Therapeutic purgation for removing excess Pitta — good for dealing with anger;

3) Therapeutic enemas for removing excess Vata — treats fear, anxiety, insomnia, tremors, nervous system disorders;

4) Nasal cleansings that clear toxins from the head — good for headaches, allergies, insomnia;

5) Blood-cleansing for removing toxic blood, generally anti-Pitta.[62]

For these procedures to work properly, the doshas must first be brought to the sites from which they can be eliminated from the body: Kapha to the stomach, Pitta to the small intestine and Vata to the large intestine. This requires a period, generally a minimum of seven days, of daily oil massage (snehana) and steam therapy (svedana). Oil massage and steam therapy loosen up the toxins in the deeper tissue and allow them to flow back into the gastrointestinal tract for their elimination. Pancha Karma is available at a number of Ayurvedic clinics throughout the United States. It can be sought out by those requiring such deeper cleansing.

13. Subtle Therapies:
Colors, Gems and Aromas

In the next chapter the most important sensory treatments of Ayurveda will be introduced. As the mind is fed by sensory perception, by altering our sensory inputs we can change our mental and emotional condition. Try some of these suggestions for yourself and see how you can improve what you think and feel simply through opening up to different sensory impressions.

Color Therapy

What would life be without color? Perhaps no other sensory potential so immediately affects, or we could say colors, our perception as does color. Color is a powerful tool for attracting our attention, shaping our moods and communicating our emotions. Color draws and catches the mind and orients it in a particular direction. Color therapy is one of the main sensory therapies for all mental and spiritual healing. It is the basis of gem therapy, which directs color on a subtle or occult level. Colors can be combined with mantra, geometrical forms and other sensory therapies for added effect.

We take in color through the light absorbed through the eyes. Color provides nutrition for the mind and life-force, vitalizing the blood and increasing our perceptual capacity. Color is the sensory quality corresponding to the element of fire, which is why bright colors arouse our motivation or our anger. Color can be used to regulate the fire element on a subtle level, strengthening mental circulation and digestion. Color affects all the other elements and can be used to harmonize them. Life is unimaginable without color and all actions color us one way or another.

Not only do we absorb colors, we also produce colors in both body and mind. Physically, the body has its pigmentation and complexion that reveals our state of health. In the disease process, discolorations arise on the skin like jaundice, pallor, skin rashes, or black or brown spots. Similarly, the mind when disturbed produces discolorations of various types. These may be bad dreams, wrong imaginations, or general disharmonious emotional tones like anger, anxiety and attachment. Countering these internal discolorations with the appropriate harmonious colors returns us to health and well-being. The wrong colors derange mental activity and the right colors restore it.

Colors and the Biological Humors

The simplest way to use color therapy is relative to the three biological humors. In this regard, colors are like spices, which also predominate in fire.

Vata

Vata does best with colors that are warm, moist, soft and calming, opposite in qualities to its cold, dry, light and hyperactive nature. This is accomplished by combining warm colors like gold, red, orange and yellow with moist and calm colors like white or whitish shades of green or blue.

Excessively bright colors, like flashy yellows, reds or purples aggravate the nervous sensitivity of Vata types. Too strong color contrasts overstimulate Vata, like red versus green or black. Too many dark colors like gray, black or brown devitalize Vata, although under certain conditions they may help ground it. Iridescent or rainbow colors, as long as they are not too bright, are very balancing for Vata. Colors for Vata are best given in shapes and textures that are round, soft, square or balanced, not thin, narrow, rough or harsh. Generally Vatas do better with more color in their lives.

Pitta

Pitta does best with colors that are cool, mild and calming, opposite its hot, light and aggressive tendencies. These are primarily white, green and blue. Pittas should avoid colors that are hot, sharp or stimulating, like red, orange and yellow.

However, very bright colors, like neon tints, tend to derange Pitta, including too much green or blue. Pittas do best with mild shades, like pastels, or with neutral colors like gray or white. Pitta types do well having less color around them or by the absence of color. For example, meditating upon the dark night sky with the stars is good for them. Yet they should avoid jet black color, although gray is fine. Pitta types should avoid colors in angular, sharp and penetrating forms and angles. They need round, soft shapes. They generally do better being more restrained in their use of color.

Kapha

Kapha does best with colors that are warm, dry and stimulating to counter its properties of coldness, dampness, heaviness and lack of movement. Kapha types do well with bright shades and strong color contrasts. They do best with warm colors like orange, yellow, gold and red.

They should avoid too much white or white shades of cool colors like green or blue, but can use these (except white) in brighter or more lucid hues.

Rich shades, like rich foods, derange Kapha. For Kapha types, colors should be bright, clear and transparent, not deep or dark. Colors which are sweet should be avoided, like pink or baby blue. Angular and pyramidal shapes are good for Kapha, which should avoid round or square forms. Kaphas do better with more color as long as it is light and luminous.

Colors and the Gunas

Not only does the specific color matter, its quality according to the three gunas must be considered as well. This factor is important for psychological conditions because color affects mental nature more directly than it does the biological humors. While color is a helpful heal-ing substance, it should not be used in excess. It can ener-gize, but it also easily becomes disturbing because its basic quality is Rajas. All colors should be Sattvic in nature: subtle, pleasant, harmonious, mild and natural. Such mod-erate use of color has a soothing effect and does not agitate us.

Rajasic colors are bright, loud, flashy and artificial, like neon signs. Their shades are bright, penetrating or metal-lic. Their contrasts are excessive, like combinations of opposite colors such as red and green or blue and yellow. Rajasic colors overstimulate and irritate the mind and senses. They should be used with discretion, particularly to counter Tamasic conditions.

Tamasic colors are dull, dark, turbid, murky, like a stagnant green or simply too much gray or black. They make the mind and senses heavy, congested and inert.

They should be avoided except for short term usage for people who are too hyperactive (have too much rajas).

White itself is the color of Sattva, whose nature is purity. Red is the color of Rajas that is dominated by passion. Black is the color of Tamas which is under the rule of darkness. However, all colors have shades that can belong to any of the three gunas. In addition, their combinations may produce an effect that can increase any guna.

Color and Tejas

Colors work particularly on Tejas, the vital essence of fire, which gives warmth, courage, fearlessness, compassion, insight and intelligence. Bright colors increase Tejas; dark colors reduce it. Colors which are too bright overstimulate and cause it to burn up Ojas, making us passionate, angry, irritable or overly critical. The right use of colors balances Tejas and keeps us clear and focused in our action and perception.

One of the easiest ways to increase Tejas in its Sattvic qualities is to meditate upon a ghee flame or a golden light. Tejas relates specifically to the saffron color (the color of the robes worn by Hindu Swamis) and can be stimulated by that as well. Excess Tejas, like conditions of anger, can be alleviated by the use of white or deep sky blue.

Application of Colors

Color therapy can be applied through an external color source. It can be visualized internally in the mind, which may begin with contemplation of the color externally. Color lamps can be made by placing colored glass over a light bulb. A soft light is preferable, avoiding florescent bulbs or neon colors. The color shades should be mild and harmonious. The body as a whole can be bathed in light of the particular color or we can bathe a specific part of the body, like putting an infectious sore under a dark blue light. For this purpose, smaller lights can be made or lamps that allow both wide and narrow focus.

Color can be applied through the clothes we wear, the colors in our house, and those in our environment. The colors used in a meditation room are particularly important. We can open ourselves to the colors in Nature, like meditating upon the blue sky or blue water, white snow or the white light of the moon, or green trees and grass. We can meditate upon flowers of different colors: the white lily, the red rose or hibiscus, the yellow chrysanthemum or sunflower, the blue iris. The harmonious shape of flowers aids in the effect of color. We can meditate upon various forms of colored glass, art works, mandalas or illuminated manuscripts. We can meditate upon fire and its various colors or do various fire rituals (homa or agnihotra).

The general rule is that impressions gained through natural sources are preferable to those gained by artificial means.

Color therapy works better when we visualize the colors in our own minds. We can then direct colors to various parts of our body, different chakras, or to our mental and emotional environment, like surrounding ourselves with a golden light.

Color therapy must be applied over a period of time for it to have a significant effect. Exposure to external color sources should be done fifteen minutes a day for a period of a month to have the proper effect. Visualization and meditation on specific colors should be done for a similar period of time. At the same time, we should avoid expos-

ing ourselves to disharmonious colors and impressions,
like the Rajasic and Tamasic colors of television and
movies.

Gem Therapy

Gems are more than wonderfully beautiful creations of
Nature. Their beauty reflects a subtle power and a connection with the mind and astral body. Vedic sciences afford
great importance to gems, particularly for their healing
and energizing properties. Gems can be used long-term to
protect and vitalize both body and mind. They strengthen
our aura and align us with the healing forces of Nature.
Though Ayurveda uses gems,[63] in the Vedic view gems are
understood primarily through astrology.

Astrology and Psychology

Astrology has traditionally had a medical and psychological aspect. Vedic astrology is used along with Ayurveda for healing the mind. The astrological birth chart
reveals the nature and destiny of the soul, not merely the
state of the body or ego. The astrologer must also deal with
psychological issues. Knowledge of Ayurveda can aid in
this process.[64]

Vedic astrology employs the same language as Ayurveda, with the gunas, doshas, elements and functions of the
mind. Vedic astrology can provide a good prognosis of the
development of psychological problems, as well as suggest
astrological measures (like mantras, gems, rituals and
meditations) for countering them. Medical astrology is a
subject in itself.

In Vedic astrology, gems are correlated to the planets
and used to balance their influences in the treatment of
physical, mental and spiritual disorders. Gem therapy is

the main method of astrological treatment. Gems are worn externally as rings or pendants. According to the Vedic system, the fingers of the hand and the planets correspond.

Index finger ....Jupiter

Middle finger ....Saturn

Ring finger..............Sun

Little finger ....Mercury

By wearing gems relating to the planets on the appropriate fingers, we can strengthen their influences. For those planets not ruling a finger, the finger ruled by friendly planets can be used. Venus is a friend of Saturn and Mercury. The Moon is a friend of the Sun and Jupiter. Mars is a friend of the Sun and Jupiter. It is always best if the gems are set so as to actually touch the skin.

Gem preparations can also be ingested internally for similar purposes in Ayurveda. However, for internal usage, gems are specially treated by complex processes to render them safe and non-toxic to the physical body. Gem preparations are used in Ayurvedic medicines today. While they are not available in the United States, we can take gem tinctures that do not actually involve ingesting the mineral.

Gem tinctures, like herb tinctures, are prepared by soaking the gem for a period of time, generally about two weeks, in a 50-100% alcohol solution. Hard gems like diamond or sapphire can be soaked for one month (from full moon to full moon). Soft, usually opaque gems, like pearl and coral, are soaked for shorter periods of time or in weaker solutions.

Planetary Colors

Each planet projects a color of the cosmic creative ray. We can also use color therapy along astrological lines to balance the effects of the planets.

Sun- ....bright red

Moon ....white

Mars ....dark red

Mercury ....green

Jupiter ....yellow, gold

Venus- ....transparent, variegated

Saturn ....dark blue, black

Rahu........................ultraviolet

Ketu ....infrared

Gems and the Planets

The classical Vedic correspondences between the major precious gems (and substitute gems) and the planets and their use as psychological remedies are as follows:

Planet	Precious Gems	Substitute Gems	Remedies
Sun	Ruby	spinel, garnet, sunstone	Self-esteem, energy, leadership
Moon	Pearl	moonstone, cultured pearls	calms mind & emotions, gives love & peace
Mars	Red Coral		strengthens will & vitality
Mercury	Emerald	peridot, green tourmaline, green zircon, jade	gives balance of mind, judgment & perception
Jupiter	Yellow Sapphire	yellow topaz, citrine	wisdom, strength, creativity
Venus	Diamond	white sapphire, clear zircon, clear quartz crystal, white coral	gives sensitivity, love & imagination
Saturn	Blue Sapphire	amethyst, lapis lazuli	gives detachment, patience & independence
North node (Dragon's head)	Hessonite garnet (golden grossularite)		gives clear perception, good judgment & sound thinking
South node (Dragon's tail)	Cat's Eye (chrysoberyl)		gives insight, focus & concentration

Uranus, Neptune and Pluto were not known to the ancients. Pluto appears to relate to dark stones like black coral or onyx. Neptune has much in common with opals, particularly the iridescent type. Uranus has much in common with the dark blue Saturn stones like amethyst.

Because most of the main planetary gem stones are very expensive, less expensive stones can be used as substitutes.

As red coral is not expensive, substitution for it is not necessary. Generally, primary gemstones require at least one carat of a good quality stone, while three carats is preferable. For secondary gemstones, three carats is minimum, five is preferable, or ten or more is good if worn as a pendant.

Use of Gems in Ayurveda

While gems have an action on the physical body, their main action is on the life-force. Not all strongly relate to one of the biological humors. Many, as subtle remedies, can help balance all three humors. We can also direct or balance their humoral action according to the metal we set them in (which serves as their vehicle). For usage in psychology, gems are long-term remedies that help balance the mind and astral field.[65]

Substitute gemstones possess the same properties as primary ones but to a lesser degree. The more expensive gem stones should be worn as rings in two or more carats. The less expensive or substitute are better in four or more (and larger stones yet can be used, particularly for pendants or necklaces).

Mineral and Gem Preparations

Ayurveda uses a number of special mineral preparations (rasas and bhasmas). These consist of various specially prepared minerals, some which are toxic in the unprepared state, for internal usage. The preparation for some minerals is relatively simple, for others it is a very complex pharmaceutical process.

These are often used for conditions involving the mind and nervous system. They include such minerals and metals as gold, silver, tin, mica, borax, iron, lead, sulfur, mercury, and gems like quartz crystal, diamond, pearl, coral, emerald, and ruby. Their use is outside the scope of this book, but they are important for Ayurvedic treatment of the mind. Metals and minerals have a stronger and more direct action upon the mind than herbs, but have to be prepared properly.

Aroma Therapy

Have you ever been upset or distressed and then happened to smell a fragrant flower or incense and noticed how your mood changed, at least temporarily, for the better? The use of fragrant oils and incense to soothe the mind and promote meditation are well known. Aromas have a great power to stimulate, calm or heal. Perhaps nothing like a fragrance can quickly change our immediate environment, affecting us down to a physical level. The right aromas promote calm and help us drop the negative thoughts and emotions that disturb us.

Aroma therapy consists of the use of fragrant oils to promote the healing process. It includes the use of incense, flower essences and essential oils. Aroma therapy is an important, though supplementary, therapy of Ayurveda, used mainly for treating the mind. It aids in concentration and meditation, calms the emotions, soothes the nerves and improves peace of mind. Here there is only the space to introduce this important subject.

Fragrance is the sensory quality that belongs to the earth element. Fragrance itself makes up the subtle earth element. Through the right use of fragrances, we can purify the earth element and open up its higher potentials, helping us forget the earthly involvements that weigh so heavily on our minds. Relating to the subtle earth element fragrances as subtle foods, we can nourish and ground the subtle body (or body of impressions). Though aromas pre-dominate in earth, they contain aspects of all the elements and stimulate all the subtle senses. The proper aromatic oils bring favorable astral influences, like those of gods and angels, into our psychic field and improve our psychic environment.

Aromatic substances have a harmonizing affect upon the mind, aid in the balance of the three humors and the three vital essences of Prana, Tejas and Ojas. They strengthen the immune system, help counter negative bac-teria and viruses, and remove stagnant air. They help clear negative emotions and astral pathogens (including nega-tive thoughts from others). They increase positive emo-tions like love, joy and happiness and strengthen our moti-vation, determination and creativity. They improve our capacity for reception, perception and discrimination.

Aromatic oils contain large amounts of Prana, the cos-mic life-force, which they impart to us. They cleanse and open the channels, allowing for the circulation of energies in the nervous system, senses and mind. They serve as cat-alytic agents to promote the right movement of the life-force on all levels. As all disease involves some disturbance or obstruction in the life-force through the Prana, aromas help treat all diseases. However, used in excess, aromatic oils can aggravate the humors (though less so than herbs).

Incense

Aromatic oils can be made into incense. This is usually the simplest method of aroma therapy and the one most common in Ayurvedic books. All forms of incense can be used for aroma therapy. Aromas derived from tree resins, barks, or branches (like cedar, juniper or sagebrush) can be burned directly or indirectly (as on charcoal for resin) as incense. Other aromatic oils require special processing to turn them into incense.

Incense can be used in various ways. We can directly inhale the incense for stronger effect or just use it to purify and beautify our air and environment. The residue from incense creates a protective film on a subtle level that lingers long after the smell has dispersed.

Some fragrant herbs can be specially burnt on different sites of the body. This is the common method of moxibustion in Chinese medicine, which uses mugwort in this way, usually burnt on a slice of fresh ginger. Ayurveda uses turmeric and calamus in a similar way. The essential oil of the plant is able to penetrate by the power of the heat.

Usage

Aromatic oils are usually applied externally. They can be taken internally but generally only if they are diluted properly. However, one should NEVER take the pure essential oil of a plant internally. A teaspoon of almost any essential oil, even mint, is enough to burn a hole in the stomach and can be fatal. Essential oils are volatile, irritating and destructive of the mucous membranes. They should not be placed directly on the mucous membranes or into the eyes.

Externally, aromatic oils can be placed on special sites on the skin. Most of these are on the head, like the third eye, the top of the head (site of the crown chakra), the temples (for headaches), the root of the nose (for sinus problems), behind the ears, or on the neck — places where they can be easily smelled.

One can put a drop of the oil on the back of one's hand or wrist and smell it periodically. The pure oil itself can be used or it can be diluted with alcohol, water or a heavier oil, like coconut or sesame. The powder of the herb may be mixed with water and applied as a paste, like sandalwood paste placed on the third eye or ginger paste on the temples.

Other important points are the heart, particularly in the center of the chest or the center of the back opposite it, the region of the chest (for lung disorders), the solar plexus (for digestive disorders or to strengthen the will), the navel, and the point of the sex center below the navel (for sexual debility). On such places we may not smell the oils, but they will affect various organs, systems or chakras by their penetrating nature. Ayurveda recognizes various sensitive points (marmas), mainly in these areas of the body, which can be treated through aroma therapy.

Internally, oils are derived indirectly from herbal teas, taken from the plant parts that contain the oils, like flowers or leaves. Essential oils can be made into alcohol tinctures, of which 10-30 drops can be taken internally with warm water. Aromatic herbs can also be taken as powders (though in powdered form their shelf life may not be very long).

Taken internally in the proper medium, aromatic oils stimulate the mind and nervous system through the tongue and sense of taste. For this reason, it is best to taste the herbs and hold them in our mouths a minute before swallowing them. In this way aromatic herbs can work directly on the Prana in the head, just as when they are inhaled.

Flower Fragrances and Spicy Oils

Aromatic oils are essentially of two basic types: flower fragrances and spicy oils. Flower fragrances, like rose or jasmine, are usually sweet in taste and cooling in energy.

Some are bitter-sweet, like jasmine or chrysanthemum. Generally flower fragrances decrease Pitta and Vata but increase Kapha. They elevate the emotions and both calm and gladden the heart, stimulating the heart chakra. They increase Ojas, the underlying energy reserve of the body and mind, though in a mild way. Many of them, like jasmine and gardenia, strengthen the immune system and in their cleansing action have natural antibiotic properties. Flowers are an important part of anti-Pitta therapy because they reduce hot emotions like irritability and anger and clear heat and fire from the head.

Spicy oils, like cinnamon or musk, are usually pungent in taste and warming in energy. They decrease Kapha and Vata but can increase Pitta. They clear the head, sinuses and lungs, stimulate the mind and senses and increase Tejas, clarity and power of perception. They improve nerve function and many are analgesic (stop pain), like camphor and mint. They help open the third eye, activate both the circulatory and digestive systems and clear the channels. Such aromas are an important part of anti-Kapha therapy.

Aromas which are purely pungent, like camphor or sage, are best for Kapha. Those which are pungent and sweet, like cinnamon, ginger or cardamom, are better for Vata. Some bitter spicy oils also exist, like wormwood and vetivert. They are good for Pitta and often possess refrigerant (strongly cooling) properties.

As fragrant oils are light and strong in smell, in excess they can aggravate Vata. They can cause feelings of light-headedness, ungroundedness and hypersensitivity. They are generally good for Vata only in the right dosage — one that is not too high.

Oils for the Three Biological Humors

VATA: Warming and pleasant oils are best, but not too stimulating. Strongly pungent oils like musk or cinnamon are balanced with sweet and calming oils like sandalwood or rose. Best oils are sandalwood, lotus flower, frankincense, plumeria, cinnamon, and basil. These are good for Vata conditions of fear, anxiety, insomnia or tremors.

PITTA: Cool and pleasant oils are best, mainly flower essences, though some cool spices or bitter aromatics are useful. Best are sandalwood, rose, vetivert, lemon grass, lotus, lavender, lily, saffron, champak, gardenia, honeysuckle, and iris. These are good for Pitta conditions of irritability, anger, or mental conflict.

KAPHA: Hot spicy oils are best. These include essential oils and resins like camphor, cinnamon, heena, cloves, musk, sage, thyme, cedar, frankincense and myrrh. These are good for Kapha conditions of attachment, depression, and mental stagnation. Sweet flowers like rose or jasmine should be avoided, as well as too much sandalwood, because these can increase Kapha.

14. The Healing Power of Mantra

Sound has a tremendous power to condition our consciousness for good or for ill. In fact, most conditioning occurs through the medium of sound, particularly as words, from which derives the education that structures our minds. Whether as words or music, no other sensory potential has such a capacity to affect us. Sound moves the mind and heart, influencing us on subconscious, conscious and superconscious levels. It can reach deep inside and touch our core desires and aspirations.

Our conditioning is nothing but the sound patterns to which we have accustomed our minds. To reprogram the mind, to remove its negative conditioning and replace it with one that is beneficial — which is the essence of psychological healing — the therapeutic use of sound is the central tool. Mantra is not only a sensory tool for healing the mind by using the power of sound and linking it with meaning and feeling, but it also affects the very nature of the mind and is part of the mind itself.

As human beings, we are primarily creatures of speech. Our words are our main means of communication and expression. The words we take in link us to the psychological patterns in others and the collective urges of society. Our words also draw up the energies and ideas latent in our psyche. Through words, our minds come together and information of all types is transmitted from which our action in life proceeds.

Sound is the sense quality that belongs to the element of ether, the seed element from which the other elements spring. Through sound, all the elements and senses can be harmonized and controlled. Sound is the basis of our bondage to the external world and also the means of freeing ourselves from it. Sound controls consciousness, which shapes itself in the form of articulate sounds or words. As ether is based upon the gross form of sound, consciousness, which is like space, consists of the subtle form of sound, which is thought or meaning.

Speech pervades all the elements, sense organs and functions of the mind. There is nothing that we contact with the mind or senses that we cannot express through speech. Speech is the very power of the mind to express itself; it is the power of knowledge to reveal what it knows. Speech pervades the universe, which itself is the manifestation of the Divine word.

Different sound formations make up the different functions of the mind. The sound vibration of impressions and information make up the outer mind (Manas). The sound vibration of abstract knowledge, principles and ideals sustains intelligence (Buddhi). The sound vibration of our deepest feelings and intuition makes up the inner mind or consciousness (Chitta). The ultimate source of sound is the spiritual heart or center of consciousness, our true Self (Atman) from which the eternal sound or Divine Word ever arises. To change our sound patterns changes the vibratory structure of our consciousness.

Mantra

There are many ways to use sound in healing, from counseling itself, which is largely verbal, to music. However, in Ayurvedic healing, the most important sound

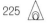

therapy is mantra. Mantra means that which saves, trayati, the mind, Manas. Mantra is the main and most direct Ayurvedic tool for healing the mind, from its deepest layers to its surface actions.[66]

Mantras are specially energized sounds or words. They may be simple single sounds like OM or special phrases or prayers intoned or sung in various ways. Mantras are repeated in a regular manner in order to empower them and turn them into tools of psychological transformation.

All conditioning through words is a kind of mantra. Any key word or phrase that we repeat, memorize and hold deep inside ourselves is a kind of mantra. When we repeat a thought of anger or hatred for another person, it is a dark or Tamasic mantra. When we repeat our desires for success and achievement, it is a Rajasic or disturbed mantra. Such mantras do not heal the mind but perpetuate its patterns of ignorance and agitation.

For truly healing the mind, Sattvic mantras, which aim at dissolving the ego and promoting self-awareness, are required. These are mantras born of love and the seeking of wisdom. Real mantra is quite different than the use of words to subconsciously influence our behavior, like advertising or propaganda, which promote ignorance and attachment (Rajas and Tamas). Mantra is not a form of self-hypnosis but a way of deconditioning the mind by breaking up unconscious sound and thought patterns through those that reflect a higher truth and energy.

Some may ask, isn't all conditioning of the mind wrong? Shouldn't we seek to decondition the mind entirely? This is a mistake and can never be accomplished. The mind, as an organic entity, requires the right conditioning, just as the body does. The body requires a specific regimen, with proper timing and manner of eating, exercise, and sleep. The mind also requires a regimen of taking in impressions, mental exercise and rest. If we fail to give the proper conditioning to the mind, we will only give it the wrong conditioning. The unconditioned is the goal, but this exists in the true Self beyond the mind-body complex. To achieve it, the mind-body complex must be put in the proper Sattvic condition first. A deconditioned mind, like an unconditioned body, will simply be out of control.

Mantra and Consciousness

Mantra means "the instrument of the mind" or "what protects the mind." Control of the mind and the unfold-ment of the hidden powers of the mind (siddhis) arise through the power of the mantra. Mantra is the main method of treating consciousness (Chitta) and is helpful for healing all levels of the mind, inner and outer. It can alter or eradicate deep-seated latencies and impressions. For this reason, it is the main Ayurvedic therapy for treat-ing psychological disorders and can be very helpful for physical problems as well.

Mantra allows us to change the vibratory pattern of consciousness. It is a direct method for dealing with the mind. Methods relying on diet, herbs, impressions, or even counseling, however useful, are indirect or external. It can be far more helpful to regularly chant a mantra than to analyze our psychological problems. The mantra changes the energetic structure of the mind which dissolves the problem, while thinking about the problem can reinforce it. Mantra changes the energy of the mental field in a pos-itive way. It is very different than analysis which, by exam-ining the patterns of negativity and how they got that way, may not alter them at all.

There is a background sound-pattern to our conscious-

ness. It may be a song we have just heard or the memory
of a painful or pleasurable event. Some movement of sound
is always going on inside us. Like the rhythm in music, it
determines the rhythm of our consciousness. The conscious use of sound can change that rhythm so that the
sound of our consciousness supports rather than detracts
from our awareness.

Our consciousness consists of deep-seated habits and
tendencies. These are the ruts in the field of our consciousness created by repeated mental activity (Samskaras).
Mantra allows us to iron them out. When we repeat a
mantra for a long period of time, this creates an energy
that can neutralize the scars left from our distracted mental activity and create a more powerful memory to override
them.

Our memories are the subtle sound vibrations that we
retain in our consciousness. Memory in the psychological
sense — the internal record of hurts and fears — is undigested sound. Such memory is misunderstood sound that
leaves a scar upon the mind. It is a vibration that cannot
be assimilated into the fabric of the mental field but
remains apart and produces changes that distort perception or lead to wrong action. Being constricted sound patterns, memories and their pain can be neutralized by the
right mantras, which project a contrary sound energy that
breaks up their stagnation.

Sound and Emotion

Any sensation we take personally, that we like or dislike, produces an emotion from fear and desire to love and
hate. Sound, as the most primary sensory potential, generates the strongest emotions. Each emotion creates a particular kind of sound. More intense emotions usually demand

stronger sounds. We sing with joy, shout in anger, cry in sorrow, groan in pain, and scream in extreme fear or pain. Those who die violently scream loudly first, reflecting the agitation of the life-force as it is prematurely cut off. Sound is a vehicle for emotion, which it can either reinforce or release.

The sound of our words carries an emotional force and transmits an emotional message. It tells how we feel and reveals our underlying psychological condition. This may be different than the actual meaning of what we say. Apparent statements of love may hide resentment, for example, or statements of happiness may hide sorrow or self-pity.

Negative emotion is nothing but a certain energy of the life-force, which is trapped by our process of self-centered consciousness. We must learn to release the energy bound up inside emotions. Negative emotions owe their existence to wrong usage of the energy of consciousness, which consists of fixing our attention on the names and forms of the external world and losing track of the greater field of existence. The release of negative emotion depends upon stopping the process that produces them. This is to reclaim our energy of attention and use it in a creative and conscious way in the present.

Mantras, through their sound energy, produce a certain emotional force or force of feeling. Through these energies we can become conscious of our emotions. Through mantra we can exercise our emotions. We can learn to play with and master emotions, which are cosmic forces of expression. We can learn how to creatively and consciously experience anger, fear, joy, or grief like an actor. We can energize them and by degrees merge them into each other, until our mind returns to its original state of pure feeling.

Mantra and Breath

Prana, the life-force, is the primordial sound vibration behind the universe. There is a sound behind the breath, which itself is unmanifest sound. Our words are created by the outgoing breath. To combine mantra with the breath is a powerful way of changing the energy of the mind. Our emotional disturbances are linked up with wrong movements of the life-force. Using mantra and Pranayama together removes these (note section on Pranayama, particularly So'ham Pranayama).

Mantra and Meditation

Most of us fail at meditation because we have not properly prepared the mental field. Meditation in the true sense, giving our attention fully to the object of our attention, requires that we already have a calm mind and controlled attention. Conditioned as we are in the modern age to entertainment, sensory indulgence and wishful thinking, this is something that we do not have. Mantra is the way to prepare the mental field for meditation. It removes the Rajas and Tamas in the mind, so that meditation, which requires Sattva to proceed properly, can occur.

Mantra provides a vehicle to carry us forward in meditation. Otherwise, distracted thought patterns disturb the mind. Mantra gives energy to meditation. To try to put the mind directly into a blank or silent state may be no more than to put our attention into our subconscious, where its dark tendencies can further inflict their pain upon us. Mantra serves like a boat to take us across the ocean of the unconscious. Mantra-prepared meditation is easier, safer and more powerful than trying to meditate directly. Once the mantra permeates the subconscious, the subconscious will support meditation, providing it far greater efficacy.

Energetics of Sound

Sounds possess specific physiological and psychological effects. Just as hot or cold weather affects our body in a certain way, so do different sounds and how we repeat them. However, the effects of external factors upon our body are easier to observe than the effects of sound. Furthermore, just as some people prefer heat while others like cool conditions, so the effects of sound, though objective, are capable of diverse subjective interpretations. Once we know the energetics of sounds we can apply them therapeutically like the use of herbs or foods.

Mantras are like Asanas for the mind. They give plasticity and adaptability to the mind. They exercise the mind's energy and give the mind poise and stability. As asana controls the body and Pranayama controls the breath, so mantra controls the mind. Mantra maintains the strength and integrity of our mental field and sustains the proper circulation of energies in it. This reduces our vulnerability to external conditioning, which, after all, is based largely on names.

Mantra therapy primarily uses what are called "bija mantras" or seed-syllables. These are prime sounds that underlie the more diverse sound patterns of ordinary speech. Though they sound simple and can be easily repeated, they are reflections of a primordial energy that cannot be exhausted.

Mantra Therapy

Mantras are the most important part of the spiritual and mental therapy of Ayurveda. Ayurveda uses mantra therapy to correct psychological and psychic disorders. Such disorders are an imbalance of energy in the mental field. A mantra of opposite energy is employed to neutralize it. Mantras are effective tools for correcting mental imbalances. They are easy to use and don't require any painful or tedious deliberation about our condition.

Mantras help balance the biological humors of Vata, Pitta and Kapha, and their subtle counterparts of Prana, Tejas and Ojas. They help harmonize consciousness, intelligence and mind. Mantras help clear subtle impurities from the nerves and subtle channels (nadis). They aid in concentration and creative thinking.

Application of Mantra

Mantras can be used by the healer to energize the healing process or by the patient to increase their own healing. Mantras can function as channels to infuse the cosmic life-force into our healing methods. They impart a spirit to the forms that we provide, allowing for a truly integral healing process.

Mantras help purify the treatment room. The mantra OM is effective for creating a healing space. HUM is good for dissolving negative energies that may exist in the treatment room. RAM can be used to bring the Divine light and cosmic life-force into the healing room. Such mantras can be chanted mentally by the healer over the client to help clear them on a psychic level. Mantras like KRIM or SHRIM can be used to energize the healing power of herbs or medicines.

For mental or nervous disorders, it is important that the patient or client chant the appropriate mantra. For example, SHAM relieves pain, tremors and mental unrest, HUM restores nerve function, counters paralysis, and

improves expression, and SOM helps rebuild the cerebrospinal fluid and nourishes the deeper mind.

Mantras must be pronounced properly, which may
require personal instruction. They must be done with care
as a sacred ritual, not as a mere pastime. To be effective, a
mantra should be repeated a minimum of a hundred times
a day for a period of at least one month. The magic of
mantra only arises after we have repeated it for some time.
Generally a mantra does not become fully empowered
until it has been repeated at least a hundred thousand
times per syllable of the mantra.[67]

Mantras can be repeated not only during meditation
but also during any time of the day when the mind is
unoccupied. It is good to repeat mantras before sleep to
promote right sleep and dreams and after waking up in the
morning to promote wholesome mental activity during
the day. Extended periods of mantra repetition can be done
like a mental fast or a clearing for consciousness. Repeating a mantra for an extended period gives a mantra bath
for the mind and clears it of any negative thoughts and
impressions. It is the best thing for cleaning the mind,
which is otherwise too dirty with its various self-centered
thoughts to concentrate on anything. A mind not cleansed
through mantra is unlikely to have the clarity for psychological peace much less spiritual growth.

Prime Mantras

OM: the most important of all mantras, it represents
the Divine Word itself. It serves to energize or
empower all things and all processes. Therefore all
mantras begin and end with OM. OM clears the
mind, opens the channels and increases Ojas. It is
the sound of affirmation that allows us to accept

who we are and open up to the positive forces of the universe. OM is the sound of Prana and the sound of the inner light that takes our energy up the spine. It awakens the positive life-force (Prana) necessary for healing to occur. It opens up all the potentials of consciousness.

RAM (with an a-sound as in 'father'): an excellent mantra for drawing down the protective light and grace of the Divine. It gives strength, calm, rest, peace and is particularly good for high Vata conditions and mental disorders, including insomnia, bad dreams, nervousness, anxiety, excessive fear and fright. It strengthens and fortifies Ojas and the immune system.

HUM: (pronounced with the 'u' sound as in our word 'put'): an excellent mantra for warding off negative influences attacking us, whether disease-causing pathogens, negative emotions, or even black magic. It is also the best mantra for awakening Agni, either as the digestive fire or the fire of the mind. It is good for burning up toxins, whether physically or psychologically, and for cleansing the channels. It increases Tejas and the perceptive powers of the mind (Buddhi) and gives control over our desire nature. It is sacred to Shiva, the God of transformation, and is the sound of Divine wrath.

AIM (pronounced 'aym'): a good mantra for improving concentration, right thinking, rational powers and improving speech. It awakens and increases intelligence (Buddhi), particularly in its creative and expressive function (Buddhi-Manas coordination). It is helpful in mental and nervous disorders for restoring powers of speech, communication, and enabling the learning process to go on. It aids in the control of the senses and mind. It is the sacred sound of the Goddess of Wisdom, Sarasvati.

SHRIM (pronounced 'Shreem'): an important mantra for promoting general health, beauty, creativity and prosperity. Shrim strengthens the plasma and reproductive fluids, nourishing the nerves and increases overall health and harmony. It gives refinement and sensitivity to the mind, helping us surrender to the truth.

HRIM (pronounced 'hreem'): a mantra of cleansing, purification and transformation. It gives energy, joy and ecstasy, but initially causes atonement and realignment. It aids any detoxification process. It is the main mantra of the Goddess or Divine Mother and grants all her blessings.

KRIM (pronounced as in 'cream'): gives the capacity for work and action and adds power and efficacy to what we do. It improves our capacity to make positive changes in life. It is good for chanting while making food or herbal preparations because it allows them to work better.

KLIM (pronounced 'kleem'): gives strength, sexual vitality and control of the emotional nature. It increases Kapha and Ojas. It grounds us and gives us balance. It also promotes artistic skills and imagination.

SHAM (with 'a' as in 'the'): a mantra of peace that can be used generally for promoting calm, detachment and contentment. It is good for mental and nervous disorders of a Rajasic nature: for stress, anxiety, disturbed emotions, tremors, shaking or palpitations. It is particularly useful in chronic degenerative nervous system disorders.

SHUM (pronounced as in 'shoe' but with the vowel not drawn out as long): increases vitality, energy, fertility and sexual vigor. Helps with the creative and artistic powers of the mind.

SOM (pronounced like 'home'): increases energy, vitality, joy, delight and creativity. It increases Ojas and strengthens the mind, heart and nerves. It is good for rejuvenation and tonification therapies.

GAM (like gum): gives knowledge, intelligence, mathematical and scientific ability, logic, verbal skills, mental stability, patience and endurance. Provides Ojas to the mind and strengthens the Buddhi.

HAUM (like owl): gives strength, power, wisdom, transcendence and transformation. Increases Prana and Tejas. It is also a Shiva mantra.

Mantras and the Elements

The five elements, and their respective sense organs and organs of action, are purified strengthened and harmonized by their respective mantras. These relate to the different chakras (see following table).

Mantra	Chakra	Element	Sense Organ	Organ of Action
LAM	Root	Earth	Smell	Organs of Elimination
VAM	Sex	Water	Taste	Organs of Reproduction
RAM	Navel	Fire	Sight	Feet
YAM	Heart	Air	Touch	Hands
HAM	Throat	Ether	Hearing	Speech
KSHAM	Third Eye		Mind-Space	Mind
OM	Head		Consciousness Space	Consciousness

In each case the 'a' sound is short, just like the vowel sound in our word 'the.' These mantras also strengthen the systems they govern.

Mantra and the Bodily Tissues

Similar mantras relate to the seven tissues (dhatus) of the physical body and can be used to strengthen them. Again the 'a' sound is short, just the vowel sound in the word 'the.' If a particular tissue is deficient, the respective mantra can be used to increase it. If a particular tissue is unstable, the mantra can stabilize it. The mantra SHAM calms the mind through strengthening the nervous system. The mantra SAM calms the emotional nature through strengthening the reproductive tissue.

1) Plasma, Air ....YAM

2) Blood, Fire ....RAM

3) Muscle, Earth ....LAM

4) Fat, Water.................VAM

5) Bone ....SHAM (as in ship)

6) Nerve ....SHAM (as in shut)

7) Reproductive ....SAM

Mantras, Shapes and Colors

Mantras can be combined with shapes and colors for added efficacy. The main shapes used reflect the five elements. Shapes along with their respective elemental forms increase the elements involved and decrease those of opposite qualities.

1) LAM   Earth   yellow square

2) VAM   Water   white crescent moon

3) RAM   Fire   red upward pointing triangle

4) YAM   Air   smoky colored six-pointed star

5) HAM   Ether   circle, dark blue in color

6) KSHAM   Mind   point, dark blue in color

For developing mental stability and emotional calm, and for promoting constructive activity, one should meditate upon a yellow square in the root or earth chakra in which the mantra LAM is resounding.

For developing receptivity, creativity, emotional harmony, and the ability to absorb positive influences, one should meditate upon a white crescent moon in the sex or water chakra in which the mantra VAM is resounding.

For developing will, aspiration, courage and vitality, one should meditate upon a red triangle in the navel or fire chakra in which the mantra RAM is resounding.

For love, devotion, and compassion, one should meditate upon a smoky gray six-pointed star in the heart or air chakra in which the mantra YAM is resounding.

For mental space, detachment, purity and wisdom, one should meditate upon a dark blue circle in the throat or ether chakra in which the mantra HAM is resounding.

For developing concentration, perception and insight, one should meditate upon a dark blue star or point in the third eye or mind chakra in which the mantra KSHAM is resounding.

Mantras and Yantras

Mantras can be used with specific geometrical counterparts called Yantras. These can be useful in psychological disorders as well. However, this is a more technical subject and there is not the space to go into it in this book.[68]

Of different yantras, the six-pointed star, combining upward and downward facing triangles, is most harmonizing. The Sri Yantra or Sri Chakra is the most complex and energizing of all the yantras. These are dealt with more specifically in the Tantric approach.

Mantras and the Biological Humors

VATA: Mantras for Vata should be warm, soft, soothing and calming. Vata types should not chant out loud or for too long as this may have a depleting effect upon their energy. After a few minutes of vocal chanting, they should chant silently.

Too much of OM is not always good for Vata as it tends to increase the space or ether in the mind, which in their case is already too high. RAM is the best mantra for them generally, as it is warming, calming and protecting.

HRIM is calming and energizing to their sensitive hearts.

PITTA: Mantras for Pitta should be cool, soothing and calming. OM is excellent in this regard, also AIM, SHRIM and SHAM, which cool respectively the mind, emotions and nerves.

KAPHA: Kapha types do well with much vocal chanting or singing. Mantras for them should be warm, stimulating and activating. HUM is excellent, also OM and AIM, which expand awareness and perception.[69]

Mantras and Consciousness

Mantras aid in all the functions of the mind.

Outer Mind (Manas)

Earth, Water and Ojas are predominant mantras, like KLIM or SHRIM, strengthen the outer mind. The chanting and singing of mantras is important on this level, as is repetition of mantra with a low voice.

Intelligence (Buddhi)

Fire and Tejas predominant mantras are good for the intelligence, like HUM or HRIM. Meditating upon the meaning of mantras brings them to the level of inner intelligence.

Consciousness (Chitta)

Air, Ether and Prana predominant mantras are good for our deeper consciousness, particularly OM. HRIM is a specific mantra for the Chitta because it helps open and clear the heart, which is the seat of Chitta. Long-term repetition of mantras is important here, particularly during sleep or idle moments during the day. Mantras reach the level of our deeper consciousness only when they go on automatically in the mind, including in the state of sleep. Mantra should follow our every breath and movement.

Caution

Mantras should be done for a spiritual and healing purpose, not to further our desires or to harm others. They require that we follow a good ethical regimen in life. After mantra, one should practice meditation. Prior to mantra it is good to study some spiritual teachings. Mantra is a tool for energizing the mind and should not be used as a substitute for real thinking or to escape our problems. It needs to be integrated into a comprehensive approach or it may not provide its full benefits.

Shiva, the Lord of Yogis

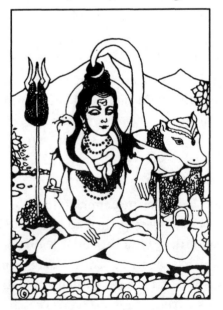

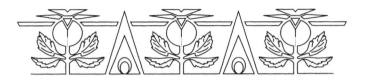

Part IV

SPIRITUAL APPLICATIONS OF AYURVEDIC PSYCHOLOGY: THE PATHS OF YOGA

Mental and emotional well-being is not an end-in-itself. It is the beginning of the spiritual life. The spiritual life moreover contains many tools to increase our psychological peace and happiness. In this section of the book, we will show how these spiritual practices are relevant from a psychological perspective. Those with a background in Yoga will find the yogic approach used and explained from an Ayurvedic perspective.

We will specifically examine the methods of Yoga and how they relate to psychology, particularly from an Ayurvedic perspective. The first chapter deals with the background of Yoga and its outer practices, its ethical foundation and its disciplines of Asana and Pranayama, yogic postures and breathing exercises. The second chapter relates to the inner and deeper practices of Yoga. Yoga in the true sense takes us beyond ordinary psychology to spiritual psychology, beyond our ordinary human problems to the ultimate problem of life — how to go beyond all suffering.

15. Spiritual Therapies

Spiritual Applications of Psychology

The psyche (mind) is rooted in the spirit (Self). Spirituality is the essence of psychology, which otherwise must remain superficial and limited. True happiness and well-being are only achieved in our inner consciousness and immortal soul, not in the ever uncertain external world. For this reason, Ayurveda always leads us to Yoga and its meditation practices. However, the term spirituality today is used vaguely and can mean any number of things. Spirituality in the yogic and Ayurvedic sense is the endeavor to unite oneself with God or the higher Self. It includes ordinary religious activity based on faith, ritual, and prayer, but only as an initial part of an inner quest for Self-realization through meditation. The spiritual life proceeds through two main factors: Devotion to God and Self-knowledge.

Devotion is the basic attitude of the soul, our spontaneous love of the Divine Father and Mother of the universe. The pursuit of Self-knowledge is the highest orientation of intelligence, the seeking to know our true nature apart from our changing outward identities. Of these two factors, devotion is more important because it is the foundation for Self-knowledge, which otherwise remains merely personal or conceptual. The practice of devotion is the nectar that can cure all ills. Without it, psychology is dry, personal and intellectual. With it, psychology becomes art, joy and wonder.

Devotion and the Place of God

How can there be a system of healing that does not recognize God and work to improve our relationship with our Creator? Ayurveda stresses the importance of God (Ishvara), the creator or cosmic lord from whom this universe springs as the ultimate source of healing. God is the manifest aspect of the Godhead or Absolute (Brahman) which rules the time-space creation. In the Vedic view, God is an inner reality, our own inner guide. Contacting him is the key to contacting our inner Self and source of well-being and happiness.

God as the Supreme Being is obviously not limited to any particular form. God is not merely "He." He (Ishvara) is also She (Ishvari). His feminine counterpart is his creative and saving power, Divine grace or Shakti. God is not only both male and female, but also animate and inanimate, existing in all of nature, including animals, plants, rocks, planets and stars. He is both personal and impersonal, formless and contained in all forms.

God is the being who works through Cosmic Intelligence, which is his mind. He respects intelligence and is ever open to our communication and our questions. The way to contact him is through meditation with an open mind and heart. As long as we exist in the realm of manifestation we are under his laws and should do homage to him. Attuning ourselves to his will lifts us to the summit of the natural world from which we can easily access transcendent awareness. The Divine will is the will to truth and for the development of consciousness. It aids all beings in their inner unfoldment regardless of the names and forms this development takes.

Importance of Devotion

Most psychological problems are based upon a lack of love in life. Love is the force that makes life worth living, gives it color, depth and warmth, allows us to feel intensely and makes us supremely happy. Love depends upon relationship. We are all seeking happiness through relationship. To be isolated causes pain. To be related and united with others brings joy. However, when we limit or personalize our relationships, they cause isolation and bring suffering. We unite with one person or group and separate from others, who become our enemies.

Desire is a state of want, a wanting to be loved. It is an empty, needy state, seeking to be filled from the outside. Love is a state of fullness, a capacity to give. It is a full and overflowing state that derives its power from within and transcends our contact with any particular human being. The real question we should ask ourselves is not where to find love, but how to give love. If we strive to give love, then love must come to us because we are looking at love as something inherent within us. If we look for love on the outside, then love must run away from us because we are looking at love as something that does not already belong to us.

Most of us seek love from the outside: from sexual partners, family and friends. We are looking to be loved in a personal way rather than to be loving in a universal way. This puts love in the distance, in some object or person different from ourselves whom we must win over in order to get them to love us. We must ever pursue love but can never keep it. Such love eludes us because it is not intrinsically ours but depends upon the circumstances of our relationships, which are ever changing.

The reason our human relationships are such a problem

today is that we are lacking in devotion. We are looking for a fulfillment in relationship with our fellow creatures that is only possible through a relationship with the Divine. Our real relationship, which is eternal, is with the Divine. Our human relationships are only temporary formations of this deeper relationship. Unless we have the proper relationship with the Divine, with the universal consciousness or truth, we will not be able to relate properly with life or with ourselves.

There is a seeking today for primary or lasting relationships. All our human relationships are secondary because they are bound by time and must pass away. They only become primary relationships when we see God within the other. Without a recognition of the eternal Being behind all relationships, there can be no fulfillment in any relationship. We are born alone and die alone and can never be one with another physically or mentally, except for brief moments.

Yet we are never really alone. Though we are born and die in a single body, there is within us the consciousness of the entire universe, should we choose to look within. We can find all worlds and all beings inside ourselves. Real relationship is to see the Divine in others and in all life. It requires that we relate to our real origin, our real parents, the Divine Father and Mother of the universe, and not just to external bodies and forms.

Lack of devotion is the root of all psychological problems. On the other hand, a person who has devotion cannot have psychological problems of a significant nature because the Divine is never absent or lacking, never apart from them.

Surrender

We cannot through our own personal power solve our psychological problems. Our willful efforts to control life and manipulate our destiny has brought us into the state of stress and agitation from which we are seeking relief. If we could have solved our problems ourselves, we certainly would have done so long ago. Nor is it of great importance to figure out the details of our psychological problems. Selfishness, which is lack of devotion, and the seeking for love externally leave us dry and discontented inwardly.

We must learn to surrender our personal problems, then they cannot cling to us. Our personal problems are merely manifestations of the personal self. There is no solution for them within the realm of the personal self. Only by giving up this self can the problems caused by it go away. Surrender is the key to this. After all, we are not responsible for how our bodies work, for the movement of time, or the marvelous order of the universe. Were there not a higher guiding power, we could not even breathe. So let us stop pretending that we are in charge of things or have the capacity to change them. Let us surrender to the Power that is always in control of things, which is the love that lies in our own deepest heart.

Surrender is the quickest way to go beyond all our problems. Yet this is not surrender to a person or belief. It is surrender to the inherent beneficence and consciousness of life that we all sense when we are free of selfish motives. Such surrender wins all things. However, surrender generally requires a form. We may have to surrender to the Divine through the medium of a friend, a teacher, or a form of God. The Hindu greeting "Namasté" itself means "I give reverence to our surrender to the Divine in you."

Compassion

Devotion and compassion are two sides of the same higher feeling capacity which is the right usage of emotion. We should feel devotion to the Divine and to those individuals who embody divine qualities, like our spiritual guides. We should feel compassion for all creatures, particularly those who are less fortunate than we are.

Compassion, however, is not pity, which is a debilitating and arrogant emotion. Compassion is feeling together or having a common feeling, regarding the other as oneself. It is not merely trying to help others, but recognizing that the sufferings and joys of others are also our own.

Without compassion for other creatures, devotion to God may become a personal fantasy. To be devoted to God means to feel compassion for all creatures, including those who may worship God differently or may not worship God at all. Compassion is a recognition of the Divine presence in all beings. On the other hand, without devotion, compassion tends to become arrogant. We as individuals cannot save the world, particularly if we have not already saved ourselves. To try to help others without first knowing ourselves is like trying to save other people in the water while we ourselves are drowning.

Yet, at whatever stage we are at in life, we can always do service to others, recognizing the limitations of what we may know and letting a higher grace work through us. The highest form of compassion is also devotion. It is to seek the descent of Divine grace for the benefit of all.

Forms of Devotion

God or the Creator is the primal teacher, the supreme guru and also the original doctor or healer of all the universe. We can acknowledge him in whatever form we like, as he takes whatever form is dear to the individual, but we will not find inner healing without his grace.

The Divine can be worshipped in many different names and forms. In fact, we should worship God in a form personal to us or our relationship to him will not be direct. We should choose the relationship with the Divine that is easiest for us to follow — father, mother, friend, brother, sister, or beloved. The mother, being the most primary and intimate of all relationships, is generally the easiest.

God is perhaps best worshipped in the feminine form of the Divine Mother. She contains within herself all love, beauty, joy and grace. Her power works through Nature, as the great beauty and delight of creation and as the evolutionary force that causes us to seek spiritual growth. God can also be seen as the Divine Father and Nature as the Divine Mother. Nature in this regard is not gross matter but the creative intelligence shaping and guiding it.

Devotion to God is part of the seeking to know who we really are, which is God. Once we gain knowledge of our inner Self, we transcend both Nature and God (the Creator) as realities outside ourselves. We become one with the Divine and with the pure consciousness behind the universe.

Developing Devotion

The best way to develop devotion is to choose a particular form of God to worship. Devotion works easiest if it begins with the use of a form. After all, it is attachment to form that is the basis of our mind's functioning and its problems. There are certain pointers we can follow. The main thing is to have a specific form of the Divine that we worship on a regular basis.[70]

1. Choose a particular relationship to cultivate with God as father, mother, beloved or friend, as the creator, preserver or destroyer of the universe, whatever is closest to one's heart.

2. Choose a particular form to worship like Shiva, Krishna, Buddha, Christ, Kali, Tara, Kwan Yin, or the Madonna, whatever is most inspiring. Such a form may be an image of God, male or female, or that of a great teacher or avatar. The figure of a great guru or teacher can also be used.

3. Take the Divine name or mantra of the form of Divinity to repeat like Om, Ram, Namah Shiv-aya, Hare Krishna and so on.

4. Do daily rituals, offerings and prayers to this cho-sen Deity. Meditate on the Deity as your true Self.

Rituals

Rituals are important for consecrating our healing practices. They are major healing practices in themselves and part of the spiritual therapy of Ayurveda. They put us in the proper frame of mind to receive the energies of our deeper consciousness. Rituals are the basis of most devotional practices, which should, however, go beyond them to meditation.

Rituals are important in psychological treatment because they bring the body and senses of the patient into the healing process. They serve to provide positive impressions to nourish and heal the mind. Very helpful are fire rituals[71] in which psychological negativity is offered into the Divine fire for purification. Standard Hindu puja or devotional worship consists of offerings for all the five senses: a fragrant oil like sandalwood for earth, liquid food for water, a ghee lamp for fire, incense for air and a flower for ether. It is a well-organized ritual for purifying the body and mind. Rituals are the most basic devotional practices. We should offer them to God in whatever form we choose to worship. They set the stage for all other practices.

Prayer and Mantra

Prayers are supplications to the Deity for help, love or guidance. We should learn to communicate with God, who, after all, is our own inner Self. We should develop a line of communication not only with God but with all creation, honoring the Divine consciousness inherent in all that exists. We can pray to the Divine and ask for help in dealing with our psychological or physical problems. God never refuses any sincere request, though he does not respond to mere ego desires.

The Deity also possesses a name or mantra. The name is the most important factor in devotional worship. We should resort to repeating the Divine Name whenever our minds become agitated or upset. If we make the Divine Name our constant companion, nothing can really disturb us in life. We should constantly keep the Name in our minds and repeat it whenever we can. Yet we should call on the Divine without ulterior motives. God or Truth exists not for our personal benefit but for the good of all, in which our own highest good resides as well.

As a first step, we should meditate upon the form of the Deity but we should also strive to see that form everywhere. We should learn to see it in others, in the world of Nature, and in ourselves. We should begin to talk to this form and seek its guidance. We should also try to understand the form and what it means on an inner level.

Along with the form of the deities in the Hindu and Buddhist traditions, an energy pattern, yantra or mandala, like Sri Yantra (note illustration), is depicted. One can meditate upon these yantras. Also various symbols can be used.

Deities and Psychology

Modern psychology tends to look upon the worship of deities as primitive or psychologically naive, but it is actually the product of a profound spiritual psychology. Deities can energize the great archetypes and cosmic forces within our own psyche, which alone have power over the deeper levels of our consciousness, both instinctual and intuitive.

Yogic deities are personifications of the great forces of consciousness which have both psychological and cosmic counterparts. The use of wrathful deities can help us overcome anger and negative emotions, whether our own or those of others. The use of benefic or peaceful deities can help calm our minds, promote contentment and awaken our deeper spiritual and creative powers.

Hinduism employs various deities who represent the different powers of the cosmic mind. For dealing with psychological disorders in general, the main deity in Ayurveda is Lord Shiva, who is the personification of the Supreme Divinity (Mahadeva). Shiva means peace and his worship grants peace of mind. Shiva has the power to control all the negative forces in the mind and rules over all the elemental forces and shadows from the past that can disturb us. He can neutralize all negativity. We can worship him through repeating his mantra:

Om Namah Shivaya! Om, Reverence to Shiva!

We can simply repeat the name Shiva over and over again. Or we can simply repeat his seed mantra SHAM, which is the root sound of peace.

For dealing with anger, we can propitiate Lord Shiva in his form as Rudra, who controls Divine wrath. For dealing with fear, we can worship the Goddess Kali who delivers us from time and death, which is what we fear the most. For dealing with attachment, we can meditate upon the Goddess Lakshmi, who holds all beneficence as the fruit of devotion. For love and joy we can propitiate Lord Krishna, who is the embodiment of Divine love and bliss. To develop fearlessness, we can honor Lord Rama, who represents Divine fearlessness.

Ganesha, the elephant-faced God, grants powers of steady intelligence, calm thinking and right judgment. He helps develop our intelligence (Buddhi) in the proper way. Hanuman, the monkey God and devotee of Rama, grants us the power of the higher life-force (Prana) that elevates the mind and increases our devotion. All the deities of Hinduism have their psychological usage. These are only a few examples to provide an idea of their psychological application.[72]

Buddhism, particularly Tibetan Buddhism, has similar deities called Bodhisattvas.[73] The deities of many other ancient religions, like the ancient Greek, Egyptian and Babylonian, were used in a similar manner. For example, the Greek Apollo, like the Vedic Sun God, was worshipped to develop powers of intelligence, creativity and enlightenment. This is a complex subject in its own right and its importance should not be underestimated.

Formless Devotion

Some people are not attracted to any form to worship and prefer to worship the Divine as formless. One way to do this is to use a relationship with the God as father, mother, beloved or lord but without any form for it. While devotion may not require form, it is impossible without a relationship with the Divine. It also usually requires the use of various Divine names or mantras.

Another way to develop formless devotion is to revere Divine qualities like truth, love, peace, and contentment. These can be meditated upon or turned into Divine names. Whatever qualities in life we honor, those we create in ourselves.

Generally it is best to combine both form-oriented and formless devotion together because the two are complementary. To see the formless in form is the highest way, which is to see God in Nature and in humanity. Those who are devoted to God in a particular form must learn to see that Divinity in all forms. Those who are devoted to the formless Divine must also see the world in God.

Developing Compassion

Most of our personal problems disappear if we consider the greater problems of the world. Actually, none of us has any personal problems. We have only our own personal form of the human problem, which is ultimately the problem of the separate self. There are various practices we can do to develop compassion.

Do daily prayers or chants for world peace and the alleviation of suffering for all creatures, such as: "May all beings be happy. May all beings be peaceful. May all beings be free of disease. May no creature suffer any pain."

Be engaged in or contribute to some service venture, which may be educational, healing, political, or ecological.

Devotion and the Mind

Highly intellectual people often do not like devotion, which they look upon as a form of emotional weakness. However, devotion is the very sap that vitalizes the mind. If we are not devoted to anything, then the mind will be dry, empty and self-destructive. Even if we are very wise or intelligent, devotion is essential. To use a metaphor, the mind is like a wick, knowledge is the flame, but devotion is the oil that feeds the wick. Without devotion, knowledge, even spiritual knowledge, will simply burn up the mind.

Self-knowledge

True psychology, or knowledge of the psyche, means to know one's Self. But who are we? Are we merely this body, this mind, the creature of this particular birth? Is knowing ourselves knowing the particularities of our body chemistry, the pattern of our memories, our social conditioning, or something yet deeper?

All psychology is an attempt to know who we really are, but different systems of psychology have very different conceptions of the self. Most accept the validity of the ego — the I-am-the-body identity of this particular birth — as our true Self. Ayurveda looks far beyond this to our identity in changeless awareness that transcends both body and mind.

Self-knowledge means understanding the full extent of our being. This is not only the physical self but the mental self and the individual soul which persists from birth to birth. True Self-knowledge means coming into contact with our soul's purpose in incarnation. What is our soul seeking to accomplish in this life to help it along its journey toward Divinity?

Self-knowledge implies cosmic knowledge. We function through the great forces of Nature, which are also powers of our own deeper awareness. To know ourselves is to know the universe, not as a physical phenomenon but as a play of consciousness. All that we see, from beautiful mountains to criminal deeds, is an aspect of ourselves. Unless we understand these within ourselves, then we must remain ignorant of who we really are.

Self-knowledge is the highest form of knowledge. It is the basis of all other forms of knowledge. It is the one thing through which everything else is known. To discover it we must take the mind back to its origin and reeducate it to see the world not as an external reality but as an internal revelation. The outer world exists for inner experience and Self-knowledge. When we approach anything in Nature directly, with a clear mind, we find that on the deepest level it is intrinsically one with our own consciousness. We see ourselves in Nature and Nature in ourselves. This is the revelation of our greater Self.

Developing Self-Knowledge

To develop Self-knowledge we must learn to observe ourselves, which requires meditation. We must not accept the conditioned ego idea of who we are but dive deep into the mind and see how we are connected to all existence. We must trace our sense of self, the I-am, back to its origin in the spiritual heart. We must learn who we are, not merely what our name or job is, but the nature of our awareness freed from all external conditioning factors.

Thought always consists of two parts: the "I" and what it is identified with, such as "I am this" or "this is mine." The subject, or "I," is connected or identified with an object. All our problems come from the object portion, which is bound by time and space. We have a problem with being this or that, or getting this or that, but we do not have a problem in being. Being is not difficult for anyone. It is the given, the Self-existent. It is in the being something or another where problems arise.[74]

To return to the pure "I am" is the root of all peace and happiness. Psychology should help us understand the outer layers of our being, our physical, vital and mental urges, not to trap us within them, but to harmonize them so that our deeper being can come forth and function through them.

Self-knowledge requires a calm and balanced (Sattvic) mind. If we are suffering from psychological disturbances, it is generally easier to develop devotion first, or to deal with the more accessible outer aspects of our lives, like changing our food or impressions. It is unrealistic to tell someone who is undergoing a severe emotional crisis simply to meditate, be detached or contact the higher Self. They need something more practical, while steering them gradually in the direction of meditation is important. For this reason, Self-knowledge belongs more properly to the spiritual path than to psychological treatment. However, Self-knowledge is the only way to ultimately go beyond all suffering, which comes from not knowing who we really are.

16. The Eightfold Method of Yoga I Outer Practices: Dharmic Living, Asana and Pranayama

The Greater System of Yoga

All life is Yoga, which means unification. We are all striving according to our understanding to become one with the real, the good, and the source of happiness. All individual life aims consciously or unconsciously at reintegration with the Cosmic Life. We are all striving to expand our frontiers and increase our connections in order to find wholeness and peace. Yoga is not a new path to follow but a way to become conscious of the original impetus of life. Yoga is the movement and evolution of Life itself.

All psychological problems arise ultimately from a misapplication of the energy of consciousness. Instead of uniting with the eternal inner reality in which is lasting joy, we attach ourselves to transient external objects whose fluctuations bring pain. The practice of Yoga, or inner integration, reverses all psychological problems by merging the mind back into its immutable source of pure consciousness, in which resides perfect peace. For this reason, Yoga is an integral and important part of Ayurveda, the science of life, particularly for treating psychological disorders.[75]

The *Yoga Sutras*,[76] the main classical text on Yoga,

defines Yoga as "the calming of the operations of consciousness." Again, the term for consciousness or mind is Chitta, referring to all conscious and unconscious thought potentials. Calming means eliminating all the negative conditionings lodged in the mind and heart. To achieve complete calm requires control of the different functions of consciousness through intelligence, mind, and ego, along with detachment from the vital force and physical body. This is a deeper and more profound definition than the common idea of Yoga today, which may be little more than exercise or stress relief. The rules for yogic development, which can treat psychological imbalances as well, are:

1) Consciousness (Chitta) must be calmed and emptied.

2) Intelligence (Buddhi) must be reoriented and sharpened.

3) Mind (Manas) and senses must be controlled and internalized.

4) The (Ahamkara) ego must be dissolved.

5) The vital-force (Prana) must be balanced and strengthened.

6) The body must be purified.

These different processes go together; without one the others cannot succeed. We have discussed these factors in different chapters of the book. In this chapter we will summarize and deepen them.

1. Calming our Deeper Consciousness

Our deeper consciousness holds the various emotional traumas and pains that disturb us, most of which remain hidden or repressed. These disturbances must be calmed and released. Peace must be brought to the core of the mind. This requires emptying the mind of its contents, its deep-seated habits, tendencies and attachments, surrendering fear, anger and desire on all levels. However, the mind is naturally calm and pure. We need only allow the mind to return to its natural state, which is to keep it free from disturbing external influences.

2. Reorienting and sharpening our intelligence

Intelligence must be redirected from its orientation to the outer sensory world and focused on the inner world of consciousness. We must learn to discriminate the eternal from the transient, the real from the unreal, our true Self from the mass of ego appearances. This requires perceiving the three gunas, holding to Sattva and discarding Rajas and Tamas. It is a key to emptying out consciousness as well. Only through the reorientation of intelligence can we direct our awareness beyond the contents of consciousness, which are all bound by time.

3. Controlling the mind

We must control our mind and senses and no longer be pulled outwardly by them to seek fulfillment externally. This requires the cultivation of self-control, character and will-power. As long as the mind brings external impressions into consciousness, consciousness cannot empty itself out. Similarly, as long as we are looking outward through the mind, we cannot redirect our intelligence within.

4. Dissolving the ego

The root of all expansion of consciousness lies in dissolving the ego or sense of separate self, which is limiting

and isolated. The separate self creates an internal empti-
ness that we seek to fill with external involvement. It causes wrong judgments through which we create pain and
suffering. As long as we are caught up in the ego, we will
not be able to control our minds, our intelligence will
remain externalized, and our inner consciousness will
remain in turmoil. This requires self-abnegation, surrender to God, and the awakening of our inner self and soul
sense.

5. Balancing and Strengthening the Vital-Force

Our Prana or life-energy becomes bound by the attachments and involvement that disturb us. To free the mind,
this Prana must be released as well. Our vital force (Prana)
must be freed from its fixation on external objects, which
fragments and disperses it. Otherwise our minds must be
drawn outward and our energy of attention lost. Without
the proper vitality we cannot do anything, and certainly
cannot control the mind and senses. This requires connecting with wholesome inner and outer sources of vitality through mind, senses, breath and body.

6. Purifying the Body

The body must be cleansed of toxins and excesses of the
biological humors of Vata, Pitta and Kapha. A toxic or
weak body will pull down the mind and weaken the vital
force. The body is the repository of our actions and holds
their long-term effects. We cannot ignore its role in working with the mind or our deeper consciousness.

Eight Limbs of Yoga: Ashtanga Yoga

Classical Yoga provides an eightfold approach (Ashtanga) to achieve its aim of reintegration. These eight "limbs" are not simply steps or stages, though they do follow a certain sequence. They are like the limbs of the body or parts of a house. Each has its proper role, though not all are equally important. We will examine the eight limbs of Yoga as psychological treatments and show how the various therapies discussed in the book relate to them.

THE EIGHT LIMBS OF YOGA

1. Yama — Rules of Social Conduct

2. Niyama — Rules of Personal Conduct

3. Asana — Physical Postures: Right Orientation of the Physical Body

4. Pranayama — Breath Control: Right Use of the Vital Force

5. Pratyahara — Control of the Mind and Senses

6. Dharana — Concentration: Control of Attention

7. Dhyana — Meditation: Right Reflection

8. Samadhi — Absorption: Right Union

The first two steps (Yama and Niyama) make up the ethical foundation of human life, the principles of social and personal conduct. Without these we will not have the right foundation for wholesome growth. They constitute the basic rules of "Dharma" or right living.

The first five steps (Yama, Niyama, Asana, Pranayama and Pratyahara) are called "outer aids" in the YOGA SUTRAS. They harmonize the outer aspects of our nature:

behavior, body, breath, senses and mind. The last three steps (Dharana, Dhyana and Samadhi) are called "inner aids." They are the central part of Yoga as embodied in the process of meditation. Together they are called Samyama or concentration, the ability to become one with the objects of our awareness. However Pratyahara can be included with the inner aids and we will do so in this book.

The Dharmic Foundation of Human Life

According to the Vedic sages, life must be based upon Dharma for us to achieve anything real or lasting. Dharma is the natural law at work behind this conscious universe. Dharma includes our social Dharma, or social responsibilities, and our individual Dharma, our personal responsibilities. Discovering our own Dharma means learning what is appropriate for us individually according to our role in society, stage of life and spiritual development.[77] Dharma is the foundation necessary for Yoga to proceed in a genuine way.

Yama — the First Limb of Yoga

Many people in the West consider that Yoga is a personal thing or even a self-preoccupation. Actually, Yoga in the true sense requires a high sense of social responsibility and ethical behavior defined by the five Yamas or rules of social conduct. The Yamas are the five main attitudes necessary to establish a right relationship with the external world.

1) non-violence (ahimsa)

2) truthfulness (satya)

3) control of sexual energy (brahmacharya)

4) non-stealing (asteya)

5) non-possessiveness (aparigraha)

The first and most important of the Yamas is non-violence: not wishing harm to any creature in thought, word or deed. Non-violence is the most important attitude for bringing about a right relationship with the world and preventing negative energies from entering into us. Violence is the greatest distorting factor in life. Wishing harm to others is the prime cause of mental unrest because it introduces an energy of violence in the mind where it must breed distortion and result in wrong action.

Truthfulness keeps us in harmony with the forces of truth in the world around us, and removes us from the influences of falsehood and illusion. It gives mental peace and equipoise and allows us to discover what is real. Truthfulness means doing what we say and saying what we do. Lying, deceit, dissimulation and dishonesty distort the mind and lead us to wrong judgment. Non-violence and truthfulness must go together. Truthfulness should not be harsh or violent. Non-violence should not be apart from truth or it is merely appeasement or placation. We should speak the truth but in a way that is as pleasant as possible.

Sex is the most powerful energy that connects us with the world and is the main source of misconduct in life. Without controlling our sexual urge, we must run into sorrow and conflict. Control of sexual energy, the most powerful of vital forces, removes us from unnecessary emotional entanglements and builds up the internal power necessary to bring the mind to a higher level of awareness. Mental imbalances always involve some distortion of sexual energy, which is the root energy of the senses and mind. Uncontrolled or misdirected sexual energy distorts our physical and mental functions. It leads to tremendous loss of energy as well as deep-seated entanglements.

Non-stealing means not taking what rightfully belongs to others. This includes not only the property of others but their work or any credit due them. It establishes our right relationship with other people and keeps us free from envy and jealousy. Non-stealing is not just a simple matter of avoiding theft, it requires honesty about who we are and what we have done and not taking anything that is not rightfully ours. Whatever we have taken from others breeds deception that warps the mind and inhibits real understanding.

Non-possessiveness means not being possessive of external things, even that which we may acquire rightfully. It requires not feeling that we own things, but considering that we are custodians of resources that belong to everyone. This principle stands for material simplicity and not craving material comforts. Non-possessiveness gives us freedom from the world. It is a particularly important observance for the modern affluent world, where we have so many possessions and such a seeking of affluence and prosperity. What we think we own actually owns us.

Non-possessiveness does not mean that we necessarily have to give away all our possessions, but it does mean that we should not accumulate unnecessary things. Having too many things creates many worries, for which the only solution may be to give them up. There are many negative psychological consequences of having too many possessions. These include suspicion and attachment, which make the mind heavy and self-protective.

Non-stealing and non-possessiveness go together. The wrong possessions, whether material or mental, like gravity, hold us down and bind us to the objects involved.

Unless we change our material environment and our mental attitude toward it, we may not be able to change the mind. We must purify our external environment in order to interiorize the mind. Too many or inappropriate possessions create a negative psychic force that prevents our consciousness from expanding. Through such yogic observances, we will no longer create a limiting material environment around our consciousness.

If we do not have an honest, truthful and detached relationship with the world and with other people, we cannot have harmony of body or mind. Wrong social conduct is the basis of most psychological and many physical diseases. Right social conduct is an important tool for treating all disease. Before we look within to treat the mind or develop our consciousness, we must create the foundation of a right relationship with the world around us, not only in our thoughts but in our actions.

Niyama — the Second Limb of Yoga

The Yogic rules of personal conduct refer to our daily life-style practices. These are the main disciplines or regimens that we must follow in order to evolve in consciousness. The five Niyamas are:

1) contentment (santosha)

2) purity (shaucha)

3) study of spiritual teachings (svadhyaya)

4) self-discipline (tapas)

5) surrender to God (Ishvara pranidhana)

Contentment comes first. This means finding happiness inside ourselves rather than in outer involvement. As long as we are discontented and distracted, we will not have the peace and consistency to look within. Yoga is not a movement of the disturbed mind seeking entertainment, but a movement of the calm mind seeking inner truth.[78] We should cultivate contentment by cultivating inner sources of creativity and awareness. This is another key to mental peace.

Purity and cleanliness are the most basic practices that we must follow in life. We should cleanse the body through proper vegetarian diet and right exercise, and cleanse the mind through proper impressions, emotions and thoughts. Lack of cleanliness on a psychological level causes as many mental problems as not cleaning the body causes physical problems. Such mental impurities include worry, gossip, disturbed imagination and jealousy.

Study of spiritual teachings means examining teachings that help us understand who we are and the nature of the universe in which we live. For this we need a genuinely spiritual or enlightened teaching based upon the works of Self-realized sages. Spiritual teachings introduce higher thoughts into the mind and teach us a language through which we can understand our own higher consciousness. Self-study includes the repetition of mantras that help us move into our deeper mind. It is not an intellectual study but requires contemplation of what we examine. We must study great spiritual truths in our own life and character and see how we create our destiny.

Self-discipline is necessary to accomplish anything significant, whether in the creative arts, sports, business or spiritual practice. We must learn to coordinate and direct our actions in a meaningful manner toward a higher goal or ideal. This means we must be willing to sacrifice what is not useful to our goal, like superficial involvement and distractions. Self-discipline is necessary to control the mind. Yoga, like all great endeavors, requires effort and dedication or we cannot go far in it.

Lastly we should never forget to honor the greater powers of the universe. We must acknowledge and surrender inwardly to the intelligence that guides this vast cosmos, apart from which we could not even breathe. This is to honor God, the universal life, and the friends and teachers who guide and help us. As long as we are open to such help and guidance, we cannot suffer from the loneliness and alienation that causes so many human problems.

If our lifestyle does not reflect such truth principles, we are also likely to be prone to psychological unrest. However, these disciplines must be cultivated on a daily basis over time. Their results do not manifest overnight. We must build a careful foundation of right conduct in order to have stability in our life and mind. Right social and personal conduct supports the proper functioning of all aspects of our consciousness. It aids particularly in the right orientation of intelligence, but also helps control the mind and senses and purify the body. Without this Dharmic foundation, what we build in life is not likely to endure.

The Outer Disciplines of Yoga

On this Dharmic foundation we can then begin the outer practices of Yoga. These consist of reorienting the body and the life-force according to yogic principles. It consists of two parts, Asana and Pranayama, the third and fourth limbs of Yoga.

Asana — the Third Limb of Yoga

Asana consists of the performance of physical postures that release physical stress and tension. The right postures increase the vital force, which gets blocked by wrong posture, and calms the mind, which is stressed by wrong posture. Asanas also help balance the biological humors that accumulate in different parts of the body. They can target certain organs or weak spots in the body and through improved circulation promote healing in these areas.

Asana in the broader sense includes all right exercise, including more active modalities, like running or hiking. The body needs a certain amount of exercise for its proper function. Lack of, excessive or wrong physical activity can aggravate or cause psychological problems. Any psychological adjustments usually require that we change how we exercise or move our bodies.

Asana in the more specific sense refers to sitting postures for meditation, which are the main Asanas mentioned in yogic texts. For any real self-examination, we must be able to sit still and comfortable with an erect spine. This allows the ascending flow of energy through which the mind can empty itself out and open up the deeper layers of consciousness.

Specific Asanas, including non-sitting postures, can also aid in bringing up repressed thoughts and facilitate their release, if the mind is prepared to deal with them. Asana practice can aid in releasing psychological tension through releasing the physical and pranic blocks sustaining it. There is much information on Asanas in various Yoga books. We will not go into it here.

Pranayama — the Fourth Limb of Yoga

Pranayama is usually called "control of the breath" — calming the disturbed pattern of breathing which agitates the mind and senses. It includes all ways of energizing the vital force through the body, senses and mind. It is not suppressing the breath, which will only cause us to die, but development and expansion of the energy of the life-force beyond its ordinary limitations. Pranayama is an important Ayurvedic method for promoting healing on all levels.

Put in simple terms, Prana is our energy, particularly that deriving from the breath. If we do not have sufficient energy, we cannot do anything in life, even if we know what we should do. If the brain does not receive proper oxygen, we do not have the mental energy to grow and to change. We lose control of our lives and become the victims of our conditioning. Old patterns from the past dominate the mind and keep us caught in their memories and attachments. We are unable to respond creatively to the present. Ultimately, the brain grows old and atrophies, the ultimate result of which is senility.

Pranayama provides this needed energy for both body and the mind. It gives power to our thoughts and intentions so we can accomplish what we really seek. On a psychological level, it gives the energy to probe into the unconscious and release the emotional and vital (Pranic) energy tied up in it. When our brain cells are flooded with additional Prana, we easily develop the insight to face our psychological problems and find creative ways of going beyond them. On a deeper level Pranayama provides us with the energy necessary for real meditation. Without sufficient Prana, meditation may only consist of spinning in our thoughts or dwelling in a blank state of mind, in which our consciousness is not really changing at all.

There are various types of Pranayama, most of which consist of deepening and extending the breath until it leads to a condition of energized relaxation. When the breath is at peace, the life-force is calmed and the senses, emotions and mind are put to rest. The disturbed movements of our vital urges cease to trouble us with their desires and fears.

Mind and breath are linked together like a bird with two wings. Thought moves with the breath and breath, in its movement, generates thought. We cannot breathe without thinking or think without breathing. For this reason, breath can be used as a rope to tie down the mind. If we concentrate on the breath, the mind becomes internalized. It is withdrawn from the senses and its external orientation on the outer world and made to turn inward. In this way Pranayama is one of the best means of Pratyahara or withdrawal from sensory distractions.

Awareness of the breath, however, is not an end-in-itself. It is a door to the deeper levels of the mind. As the mind focuses on the breath, the deeper layers of consciousness gradually open, releasing the subconscious and all that is hidden within. As the mind draws more energy through Pranayama, deeper thoughts come up, including emotional issues which we will have to deal with through meditation or their energy will disturb us and prevent us from going deeper.

So'ham Pranayama

So'ham is the natural sound of the breath. The sound of the air coming into the nostrils produces an "ess"-sound. The sound of air pushed out the nostrils produces an "h"-sound. Observe this for yourself. The Sanskrit root "sa" means to sit, exist, hold and therefore to inhale. The root "ha" means to leave, abandon, negate and therefore to exhale. Sa means He or the Supreme Spirit. Ham means aham or "I am." So'ham is the natural sound of the breath proclaiming "I am He" or "I am the Self of all Beings."

This sound leads us beyond the mind to our inmost nature as pure awareness.

So'ham Pranayama is easy and natural. One does not try to manipulate or control the breath but merely lets it deepen of its own accord, following the sound current back to the core of awareness.

Some Yoga groups use Hamsa — using ham for inhalation and sa for exhalation — instead of So'ham. This is another version of the same approach, with the sounds reversed. So'ham works to energize the breath as it increases its normal flow. On the other hand, Hamsa works to still the breath as it counters its normal flow. So'ham is better to strengthen the breath, Hamsa to calm it.

The Nadis

The subtle body, like the physical, consists of various channel-systems called nadis, which literally mean streams. Seventy-two thousand nadis exist. Of these, fourteen are significant, and three are important for all yogic practices.

Sushumna: Most important and central of the nadis is the Sushumna, which corresponds to the central spinal canal in the physical body. It controls all the functions of the chakras that are strung like lotuses upon it. The chakras, in turn, rule over mind-body functions in their ordinary function. In their awakened or opened condition, they bring about the unfoldment of higher states of consciousness and superconsciousness. The Sushumna is called Chitta-Nadi in yogic literature, [79] the channel of the Chitta or deeper consciousness. It is the energy flow of the entire mental field itself, the stream of consciousness.

Bringing our Prana and attention into the Sushumna is the key to calming the mind. Sushumna has the nature of ether and is balanced in terms of the biological humors and Pranas. The Kundalini, or Prana Shakti, which is fire (Tejas) predominant, activates it. Placing the united energy of the breath, senses and mind into the Sushumna arouses the Kundalini. This requires tremendous concentration and detachment in order to so gather our energies. It should never be attempted willfully or forcefully but as part of a process of deepening inner peace and equanimity. Kundalini is the force for developing higher levels of consciousness. To deal with it properly requires the proper foundation of Yamas and Niyamas first.

Ida and Pingala: Left and right of the Sushumna run two major nadis, whose movements intertwine like a series of figure eights put one on top of the other as in a caduceus. These start at the base of the spine and move from side to side, chakra to chakra. The left nadi ends at the left nostril, the right nadi at the right nostril. These two nadis govern all the other main nadis and are responsible for the left brain/right brain predominance. The left or lunar nadi dominates right brain activity that is feeling-oriented. The right or solar nadi dominates left brain activity that is rationally-oriented.

The Ida is the left or lunar nadi that has the energy of the Moon. It is white in color, feminine, has a watery (Kapha) nature, is cool, wet and soothing. Ida literally means food, refreshment, and inspiration. It operates more during the night and promotes sleep and dreams. Physically, the Ida sustains the tissues of the body that are water (Kapha) predominant. Psychologically, it promotes emotion, sensation and imagination — the functions of the outer mind.

The Pingala, which means red, is the right or solar nadi and has the energy of the Sun. It is masculine, has a fiery

(Pitta) nature, is hot, dry and stimulating. It operates more during the day and promotes wakefulness and activity. Physically, the Pingala governs digestion and circulation. Psychologically, it promotes reason, perception, analysis and discrimination — functions of intelligence (Buddhi).

These two channels, in an opposite way, relate to the right and left hemispheres of the brain. People who are dominated by the right hemisphere have the feeling and intuitive potential of the Ida, the left lunar nadi. People who are dominated by the left hemisphere have the rational and critical potential of the Pingala, the right lunar nadi.

The breath flows primarily in one of these two channels, alternating every few hours according to factors of time, environment, age and constitution. We can determine the physical and psychological condition of a person through observing the nostril in operation at any given time. When the right breath prevails, the masculine, fiery, aggressive or rational side of our nature predominates. When the left breath prevails, the feminine, watery, receptive and feeling side of our nature has ascendancy. When the Prana or life-force is balanced and the energy in the solar and lunar nadis equalized, the mind is brought to a peaceful state of heightened awareness.

Just like the channels of circulation in the physical body, the nadis can be disturbed by wrong flow of energy through them. Excess flow through the solar nadi brings about hyperactivity of mind and body. Psychologically it causes excess clarity, anger, critical disposition, and manipulativeness (Tejas derangement). Physically it causes insomnia, dizziness, fever, and hot sensations in the head (Pitta derangement).

Excess flow through the lunar nadi brings about emotional vulnerability, disturbed imagination, and domination by astral forces. Physically it causes excessive sleep and dreams, congestion and unusual weight gain (Kapha derangement).

The flow in the nadis is disturbed by negative emotions, egoism, poor intake of impressions, and poor mental digestion. Physical factors include wrong diet, particularly too heavy or greasy foods like meat, cheese, sugar or oils, lack of exercise, shallow breathing and excess sex. Suppression of emotion is the main factor for blocking them. Drugs or forceful exercise, breathing or meditation practices are additional aggravating factors. Such things create toxins that hinder or block the flow of energy in these subtle channels.

Alternative Nostril Breathing

An important key to mental and physical health is to keep the nadis clear and maintain a balanced flow between the Ida and Pingala. It also helps balance Prana, Tejas and Ojas and treats the mind and emotions. Meditation, mantra, the right intake of impressions, physical remedial measures like Asana, bodywork, herbs and diet help clear the nadis. Pranayama, however, is the main method, particularly alternate nostril breathing, which is called nadi shodhana or "cleansing of the nadis."

Since the left nostril is lunar or Kapha predominant, promoting the breath through it increases our bodily tissues, Ojas and gives nourishment to the outer mind (Manas). Left nostril breathing counters fever, insomnia, anxiety, anger, hyperactivity, and hypersensitivity. Cooling or lunar Pranayama is best for Pitta constitutions and their problems of excessive heat and agitation.

Since the right nostril is solar or Pitta predominant,

promoting the breath through it increases Tejas, courage and motivation, and Buddhi (intelligence). Right nostril breathing counters poor digestion, poor circulation, lack of motivation, depression, laziness, and paralysis. It is good for Kapha problems of excessive weight and attachment.

Increasing the breath equally through both nostrils calms Vata, increases Prana and harmonizes our deeper consciousness (Chitta). It counters Vata conditions of fear, anxiety, indecisiveness, and confusion, but in order for it to be effective we should practice it along with a rich, nutritive diet and proper intake of oils and fluids. Pranayama aids in the conversion of food and water, which helps Vata constitution put on more weight and nourish the nervous system, but it must be combined with proper food and water to do this.

17. The Eightfold Method of Yoga II Inner Practices: Meditation, Samadhi and the Transformation of Consciousness

We are all seeking unqualified happiness and enduring peace in life. Only this can bring fulfillment to our minds and hearts. Yet whatever we achieve in the outer world is never sufficient, however good our relationship, career success or intellectual attainments may be. We are ever seeking something greater, something pure, perfect or sacred, not touched by the fluctuations and imperfections of time and circumstance. Yoga teaches us how to realize this. We will examine this inner secret of Yoga in this chapter.

The inner practices of Yoga consist of the four higher levels of yogic practice: Pratyahara, Dharana, Dhyana and Samadhi — withdrawal from the senses, concentration, meditation and absorption. On this level we are working directly with the mind itself, down to its deepest core level in the heart. This is only possible from the foundation of the earlier stages of Yoga, an ethical lifestyle (Yama and Niyama), control of the body (Asana) and control of the breath and vital force (Pranayama). Through this foundation we can gain access to those mysterious corners of the heart in which both our sorrow and joy are hidden and can be understood.

Pratyahara — the Fifth Limb of Yoga

Pratyahara is perhaps the least understood aspect of Yoga and yet the most important for any psychological treatment. It is often translated as "withdrawal from the senses." More accurately it means "withdrawal from distraction," which means detaching the mind from the impulses deriving from the senses. Distraction is our vulnerability to external stimulation, our capacity to be conditioned by environmental forces.

Each sense organ has its own urges, its built-in programming. Each is like an unruly child demanding our attention and seeking gratification. Each sense organ colors the mind and tries to impose its likes and dislikes. The eye-consciousness urges us to seek pleasurable and avoid painful visual sensations. The vital force or Prana in the eye drives us to promote actions that provide visual sensations. The ego operating through the eye tries to keep our attention in the eye and make visual sensations the most important part of our self-identity. It is the same with other sense and motor organs.

The motor organs, particularly the speech and reproductive organs, are harder to control than the sense organs. The motor organs have a greater vital force and more urgency to their expression. They have a more active nature that demands more attention. Yet the motor organs only express what comes into them through the sense organs. We can also control the motor organs through control of the sense organs.

Without the proper control of the senses, the mind becomes fragmented in five directions. Sensory fluctuations, which can be very major, keep the mind off balance and can lead to psychological problems and loss of self-control. As long as we are dominated by the senses, our

sense of gravity lies outside ourselves and we have no internal stability or strength of character. We become a creature
of the moment and react to whatever happens around us.

Pratyahara is control of the senses, which includes right
management of impressions. It means keeping our mind
aloof from the senses and in control of their input. It is not
suppression of the senses but their right application, which
is as instruments of perception rather than as the judges of
what we perceive. According to Ayurveda, all diseases arise
from wrong use of the senses, which may be excessive,
deficient, or improper. How we use our senses determines
the kind of energy we take in from the external world,
from food to emotion. Pratyahara includes all the sensory
techniques of Ayurveda, particularly those we have discussed under right use of impressions, color and mantra
therapy.

The techniques of Pratyahara are primarily of two
types: shutting off the senses, like closing the eyes or ears,
or using the senses with attention rather than distraction.
Closing the sensory openings is a practice like fasting for
the body. Fasting from impressions allows the digestive
capacity of the mind to renew itself, just as fasting from
food allows the body to cleanse itself by digesting toxins.
It also allows inner impressions to be cognized, like the
inner sounds and lights. This can be done simply by closing the eyes or staying in a dark and quiet place.

Pratyahara can also be practiced during sensory perception. This occurs when we witness sensory impressions,
when we dwell in pure perception rather than react with
likes and dislikes. It requires that we cease to project
names and definitions onto our impressions and see sensory objects for what they are, which is a play of sensory
energy. One way to do this is not to focus upon objects

themselves but upon the sensory impressions — the sounds and colors that make them up. Another way is to look at the space between objects rather than at the objects themselves. Perhaps most significant is to meditate with one's eyes open while directing one's attention within.[80]

Pratyahara can employ internal objects for directing our attention away from external objects. Most important in this regard are mantra and visualization that direct inward the energy of the senses, which is essentially sound and light. In this way we creatively use the energy of the senses on an inner level. This also helps open up inner sensory sources, the inner light and sound.

Pratyahara follows from Pranayama. In Pranayama we gather our breath and Prana. In Pratyahara we take this concentrated Prana and withdraw it from the field of the senses into the field of consciousness. We can visualize withdrawing our Prana stage by stage from our limbs, organs and mind, resting it within the heart.

Pratyahara is assisted by creating a special environment that provides different and better impressions. It may involve retreat in a secluded place, like in a mountain cabin, where the person is removed from ordinary distractions. It may involve setting up an altar or healing space in the home, which similarly removes us from ordinary impressions and develops those of a higher nature. Such a sacred space helps insulate us from vulnerability to external influences. Pratyahara methods are particularly important for individuals who are hypersensitive, impressionable, and easily influenced.

Pratyahara is the main method for strengthening the mental immune system and its capacity to ward off negative impressions, emotions and thoughts. Pratyahara is perhaps the most important aspect of Yoga for psychological disorders because it restores the proper relationship between the mind and the external world. It cuts off the reception of negative influences from the outside and opens up the reception of positive influences from within. It seals the mental field from negative energies so that healing can occur. Most of the sensory therapies of Ayurveda fall mainly in this category, such as we discussed in the right intake of impressions and the use of mantra, sound and color.

Dharana — the Sixth Limb of Yoga

Dharana is concentration or right attention, which is the ability to give all our mental energy to the object under examination. The quality of our attention in life determines our state of mind. Attention is the central pillar that upholds our mind and character and gives power to all we do.

The problem is we throw our attention away on the external world, seeking approval or enjoyment. We are not taught to control our attention but, rather, to make ourselves vulnerable to social conditioning through sex, advertising and entertainment. Most psychological problems arise from lack of attention, in which we let some outside force, or some subconscious influence, rule us. We let others tell us who we are, what to do or even what to think.

Dharana techniques consist of different methods to make the mind one-pointed, including concentration on particular objects. Some of these methods are the same as Pratyahara. In Pratyahara the goal is negative, to withdraw from sensory distraction, in which case the nature of the object itself is not important. In Dharana the goal is positive, to become focused on the particular object, in which the nature of the object can be crucial. Hence Pratyahara leads to Dharana. Pratyahara gathers the energy of the mind; Dharana focuses it.

Simple Dharana methods involve gazing at various objects like a ghee lamp, candle, statue or picture, or some object in nature like the sky, the ocean, a tree, mountain or stream. Internal Dharana methods involve focusing on inner lights and sounds, or visualizations of deities, mantras and yantras. Dharana can be done on the elements, the chakras or the gunas. A formless Dharana can be done on various cosmic truths, like focusing the mind on the impermanence of all things or upon the unity of all existence.

In psychological treatment, such attention-developing techniques can be taught to patients to aid in mind control and the development of memory. These include simple things, like concentrating on a single object or training the memory to hold a particular thought. Even mathematics or learning a language can be used in this way. They help train the mind to function objectively and remove it from the emotional subjectivity that clouds its function.

Dharana is the way in which the mind (Manas) is controlled and the inner intelligence (Buddhi) is awakened. The focused mind has the ability to establish goals, values and principles. It leads us to truth. Regaining control of the mind and being able to direct it at will is the key to all success.

Pratyahara and Dharana Techniques

The following are a few practical techniques in Pratyahara and Dharana.

MEDITATION UPON THE FIVE ELEMENTS

Ether Element: The Sky

Find an open area where you can have a clear and unobstructed view of the sky. Lie down on your back and gaze into the sky for at least twenty minutes, being careful not to look near the sun. Meditate upon your mind as being like the sky. When you return to your ordinary perception, you will find your mental field cleansed and renewed.

You can practice the same method at night, preferably a moonless night in an area where there is no interference from city lights. You can start right after sunset and gradually watch the stars come out. This takes about two hours. Or you can wait until the sky is dark and gaze at the stars continually for about twenty minutes. This will cool and calm the mind and open up higher perceptual and intuitive faculties. This meditation is best done on the ether or throat chakra and aids in its unfoldment.

Air Element: Clouds

Find an open area where you can have a clear and unobstructed view of the sky, avoiding looking at the sun. Choose a day that is partly cloudy, where you can watch both white and dark clouds in their formation and movement. Meditate upon your thoughts and feelings as being like the movement of the clouds in the infinite space of awareness. Again, take at least twenty minutes. This meditation is best done on the air or heart chakra and aids in its unfoldment.

Fire Element: A Candle, Ghee Lamp or Fire

Set up a candle or ghee lamp on an altar or special spot

in a quiet room. Gaze at the flame for fifteen minutes. Try not to blink. Let tears come to your eyes if necessary. Let your mind merge into the flame. See the outer light as your inner light.

In the case of a fire, gaze into the fire and offer your negative thoughts and feelings for purification. Let the fire purify them and expand them into a positive energy of love and joy for the entire universe. This meditation is best done on the fire or navel chakra and aids in its unfoldment.

Water Element: The Ocean, a Lake or a Stream

Find a place where you have a good view of the water. Sit comfortably and gaze at the water. Let your mind clear itself out and merge into the water, letting the mind's movements be like the movement of the waves or the flow of the stream. Do this for at least twenty minutes. It is best done on a clear day when the transparency of the water can be seen. Feel your mind as cool and refreshed, and your heart open and vibrant. This meditation is best done on the water or sex chakra and aids in its unfoldment.

Earth Element: A Mountain

Go to the top of a mountain or hill, preferably where you have a view of other hills or mountains. Sit and focus your mind on the lower slopes of the mountains and on the distant mountains and valleys. Feel the earth within you. Feel as grounded and stable as a mountain, and as open to the sky. Feel one with Nature and above all the petty problems of humanity. Do this for at least twenty minutes. This meditation is best done on the earth or root chakra and aids in its unfoldment.

OTHER MEDITATION TECHNIQUES

Particular Colors

Gaze on or visualize particular colors, like dark blue, saffron orange, gold or white. This can be combined with mantras or deities. Examine the section under color therapy for more information.

Picture of a Great Teacher or Deity

Meditate upon the picture or statue of a deity or great teacher, trying to contact its spirit and link up with its grace and wisdom. Let the figure communicate to you through the picture. Memorize the teaching given and see how it applies to you. It is important to put the mind in a silent or receptive state. Imagination should not be encouraged.

Mantras

All that has been taught about mantra is useful here. Take one mantra and concentrate the mind upon it. Repeat it first audibly for five minutes, then mutter it softly for ten minutes. Then repeat it mentally for twenty minutes. Do this morning and evening for one month and see how it improves your mental powers.

Geometric Devices, Yantras and Mandalas

Focus on a yantra, like Sri Yantra. Visualize it in your mind and memorize it. See the vibration of the mantra OM within it. Do it for at least a month like a mantra.

Inner Sounds

When you close your ears you can hear various inner sounds. Some are physiologically produced, while others spring from deeper levels of consciousness. One can concentrate on these sounds and the vibrations that come through them. Sounds occur like the ocean, a drum, a flute or other musical instrument. Listen to these sounds and try to connect with the higher forces and energies coming through them.

Inner Light

A light can be seen in the region of the third eye. It may be faint at first, whitish or golden, or like a mass of molten metal. Concentrate on this, not as an external object but as a connection to the Divine within. Let this ball of light as the power of cosmic consciousness come to you and sink with pressure into your heart.

Affirmations

Affirmations involve withdrawing the mind from its ordinary thoughts and concentrating upon a particular goal. However, we should affirm the inner truth of our being, not try to empower our ego or desire nature. We should affirm the fullness of our inner nature, not the desires of our outer nature.

For Pratyahara there are special affirmations like: "In my nature as pure awareness I am inherently free of the need for external objects and enjoyments." For psychological problems, a good affirmation is: "In my true Self I am above the mind and its problems. Let them come or go. They cannot affect me."

For Dharana there are other affirmations like: "In my true Self I am in control of my mind and can concentrate it on whatever I need to understand." Affirmations can also be a form of Pranayama, in which the life-force is increased, such as: "I am in contact with the cosmic life-force, which nourishes me and provides energy for all that I need to do."

Dhyana — the Seventh Limb of Yoga

Dhyana is meditation in the true sense, which is the ability to sustain long-term attention on the object of our examination. Dharana sets our attention on a particular object; Dhyana holds it there. Sustained Dharana in time becomes Dhyana. Generally Dharana must be continued for at least one hour for true Dhyana to occur.

Once the mind is able to focus on an object, it automatically receives knowledge of that object. Whatever we give our attention to will gradually unfold its meaning for us. Dwelling on that knowledge is meditation. Meditation is not simply wishful thinking, nor is it merely sitting trying to control one's thoughts (which is at best an attempt to meditate). Meditation occurs through sustained attention.

Meditation may be practiced with or without form; the former prepares us for the latter. Meditation with form employs the same techniques as Pratyahara and Dharana, holding the mind on a particular object, but sustained over a longer period. Any object that draws the mind can be used: a form in nature, a deity, a guru, a yantra or a mantra. Formless states of Dhyana involve meditation on truth principles, like "all is the Self," or meditation on the Void which transcends all objectivity.

Meditation can be passive or active. Passive meditation involves the mind reflecting on an object, form or idea. It creates a witnessing consciousness in which we can choicelessly observe all the movements of the mind. It provide space in which our inner consciousness (Chitta) can open up. One simply abides in the state of the Seer.

Active Dhyana consists of various forms of inquiry through which we look into the truth of things, using the concentrated mind as the instrument. Self-inquiry, such as explained in the section on Self-knowledge, is the most important active method of Dhyana. Active Dhyana activates the inner intelligence (Buddhi). Generally, active methods of meditation are stronger than passive methods, but both go together. It is easy for the mind to fall into a blank state or get caught at a certain level with passive meditation. Inquiry keeps the mind going deeper. Active and passive meditation can be combined, as when one alternates inquiry with some passive contemplation. When the mind tires of one it should be directed to the other. If the mind tires of both, it should be held to a mantra or go back to Pranayama.

The highest states of meditation involve going beyond all thought. This occurs when consciousness is emptied of its contents through the understanding of their nature and development. True meditation (Dhyana) cannot be achieved by a restless or emotionally disturbed mind. It requires properly developed concentration, which itself rests on control of the body, senses, vital force and mind. These depend upon a predominance of Sattva guna in our entire nature. For this reason, we must first purify our life and mind. Otherwise, to simply try to not think is to put ourselves in a blank state, in which our consciousness is not transformed but merely put to sleep. We should not rest content in any state of mind but seek to go to the root of who we are.

Much of what is called meditation today is more prop-

erly Pratyahara (like visualization) or Dharana (concentration techniques). Such meditation is useful for calming the
mind in psychological derangement. The stress-relieving
effect of meditation has been researched and validated in
recent years. Stress is an accumulation of tension in the
mind. Meditation, expanding the mental field, relieves it.
Such basic forms of meditation like mantra or concentration exercises are useful in psychological problems because
anyone can do them. The higher forms of meditation are
only possible for those who have already gone beyond ordinary human problems and attachments, which is not easy
in this hectic modern world.

Meditation on Death and the Deathless Self

One of the best meditations is to meditate upon death.
This is not something morbid; it is simply facing the ultimate reality of our lives. It is very healing to all our psychological problems that revolve around our transient personal problems.

Sit or lie down comfortably. Imagine that your body is
dying. Withdraw your attention from your body, senses
and mind and place it in your heart. Imagine that you are
a small flame in the heart of this great city of the body.
Offer all your thoughts and feelings into that immortal
flame. Realize that flame as the True Self, the I-am-that-I-
am. Let everything else go. Bathe, purify and transform
yourself in that pure light of awareness. See all the universe, all time and space within it.

Samadhi — the Eighth Limb of Yoga: [81]

Samadhi is the last and highest limb of Yoga. It is the
central aspect of yogic practice. In fact, Yoga is defined in
the Yoga Sutras primarily as Samadhi.[82] Samadhi is the

capacity of consciousness to become one with its object of perception, through which the nature of ultimate Reality is known. It can perhaps be best translated as "absorption." Samadhi is the capacity to merge with things in consciousness and gives ultimate joy and fulfillment in life. It is the highest stage of meditation that brings us to the underlying Divine nature in everything. It is the natural outcome of true meditation. Sustained meditation results in Samadhi.

Samadhi is also of two types: with or without form or quality, just like meditation. Preliminary Samadhis involve heightened perception, deep thinking and contemplation, and are with form or thought. Higher Samadhis involve transcending thought to pure consciousness devoid even of the highest thoughts and experiences. Yet it is very difficult, if not impossible, to reach the thought-free Samadhis without having already developed the Samadhis of deep thinking and profound inquiry. Much profound contemplation is necessary to develop Samadhi. It is not something that comes in a day or even in a year and may require decades of practice to really manifest.

To approach Samadhi in the yogic sense is not possible for one whose mind is not developed or who is suffering from psychological imbalances. Psychological cleansing must come first or the mind cannot reflect the state of Samadhi in an undistorted manner. In this regard, Ayurvedic psychology lays the foundation for yogic Samadhis.

Samadhi is the main way that our inner consciousness (Chitta) develops, which occurs through the higher function of intelligence (Buddhi). In Samadhi we return to this core consciousness (Chitta) and can perceive all its functions. Hence Samadhi helps us to understand how the mind works and how to change it. The knowledge gained from Samadhi adds much greater depth to any psychological treatment. Ayurvedic knowledge has this efficacy for treating the mind because it was originally born of Samadhi, the realization of the ancient rishis.

Lesser and Greater Samadhis

We are all pursuing Samadhi or absorption in one form or another. There are not only the higher yogic Samadhis but ordinary Samadhis. We are only happy when we are so engrossed in something that we forget ourselves because the separate self is sorrow. Samadhis are peak experiences in which we become lost in the object of our perception. Being inspired, enwrapped in music, engrossed in a movie, or lost in a sexual experience are all lesser Samadhis.

Yoga teaches that there are five different levels of consciousness (Chitta):

1) deluded (mudha)

2) distracted (kshipta)

3) imaginative (vikshipta)

4) focused or one-pointed (ekagra)

5) calmed (nirodha)[83]

Samadhis exist on all five levels of consciousness, but Yoga as a spiritual discipline is only concerned with Samadhis of the last two levels, which are purely Sattvic (spiritual) in nature. These are arrived at through the development of our higher awareness and are under the control of our deeper intelligence. They are the greater or the yogic Samadhis.

Samadhis of the one-pointed mind involve the use of an idea or support, from contemplating an object in nature to reflecting on the nature of ultimate Reality. They are focused on a particular object that may be external or internal. Here the mind consciously gets concentrated in the object and its underlying cosmic truth is revealed. Yogis use this type of Samadhi to uncover the secrets of the cosmos and the psyche.[84] These are an extension of the methods of Pratyahara, Dharana and Dhyana that we have already discussed.

Samadhi of the calmed mind is beyond all objects and thoughts and involves stilling or silencing our consciousness on all levels. This type of Samadhi is necessary for transcending the outer world and for Self-realization. Generally one must develop the Samadhis of the one-pointed mind in order to develop those of the calmed or silent mind.

The lesser or non-yogic Samadhis are transient in nature and cannot permanently bring peace to the mental field. They occur when the unpurified mind comes under the temporary domination of one of the three gunas and through this merges back into its core (Chitta), which is the level of the gunas. When one guna prevails there is an absorption in that guna. But in time the other gunas must assert themselves and the Samadhi comes to an end. These lesser Samadhis are outside the control of our awareness and depend upon circumstances. Such lesser Samadhis are the main cause of mental disturbances because they breed attachment and cause addiction to them.

Samadhis of the Deluded Mind

Samadhis of the deluded mind include sleep, comas, and states induced by alcohol or drugs in which the quality of Tamas or dullness prevails. Here the mind is absorbed in a blank state in which consciousness of the body is obscured or even lost. One loses control of one's mind and gets absorbed in a mindless or non-feeling state, or one gets absorbed in a sensation in which there is no movement, like a drunk lost in a drunken stupor lying half-conscious on the floor.

Samadhis of the Distracted Mind

Samadhis of the distracted mind occur when the mind is so engrossed in an activity or external sensation that it forgets itself. Here the quality of Rajas or energetic movement prevails. This type of absorption occurs in sexual activity, in sports — like the enjoyment of running fast — or in watching a movie (which has an element of Tamas, however, being mainly a passive sensory enjoyment). The mind is calmed by the weight or intensity of sensory stimuli. It occurs when we are engrossed in our work, which is why overwork can be an addiction. We get so lost in what we are doing that we forget ourselves. This state of mind is behind most of the ordinary achievements of life, in which we imagine a goal for ourselves and then pursue it. The attainment of such goals like wealth or fame is a kind of Samadhi experience, the absorption of success.

Samadhis of the distracted mind can occur on a negative level when the mind becomes engrossed in great fear or pain. Any intense emotion, including violence, creates a drama in which the mind becomes concentrated, a kind of Samadhi.

Samadhis of the Imaginative Mind

Samadhis of the imaginative mind occur when the mind is so absorbed in its own projections that it forgets itself. This occurs mainly when the quality of Sattva prevails. These are the Samadhis of the inspired mind or genius. Such are the visions of artists, the musings of philosophers, and the great discoveries of scientists. They include many transient spontaneous religious or mystical experiences.

While Sattva prevails in this Samadhi, Tamas and Rajas have not been eliminated and so assert themselves after a period of time. In this regard, Yoga does not look up to these creative or intellectual Samadhis as the ultimate, which is the tendency of Western intellectual culture to glorify genius as the highest human type. Yoga is based on higher Samadhis and, while honoring these Samadhis of the inspired mind, realizes that these are not sufficient to purify the mind, particularly the subconscious. They cannot overcome the other gunas of Rajas and Tamas that will again bring the mind down and cause it pain. Such inspired Samadhis are like a window on the higher Samadhis but cannot take us there. This requires more than cultivation of the intellect; it requires a yogic type training. It requires not imagination but realization.

Samadhis of a mixed nature exist in which the three lower Samadhis combine because the three gunas behind these states are ever fluctuating. Generally, Samadhis of the distracted mind lead us to a Tamasic state, when we are exhausted by them, just like the joy of running a race leads to the pleasure of deep sleep.

Lesser Samadhis include all the powerful experiences of life to which we get addicted and cause us sorrow. The mind gets trapped in the influence of such peak experiences or moments of intensity and these serve to color and distort it. Whatever experiences most impress the mind give us the greatest sense of absorption or self-loss, determine our background state of mind and the external conditions that we will create for ourselves. For example, the mind, dominated by the pleasure of sex, will promote a

consciousness and way of life seeking sex. A mind domi-
nated by the joy of artistic inspiration will seek that.
Severe mental disorders involve more powerful lesser
Samadhis.

Schizophrenia

Schizophrenia is a Samadhi of an inferior nature, generally dominated by Tamas or delusion. The person may go
into a trance, see hallucinations, hear voices or other delu-
sory sensory phenomena in which darkness covers the
mind. The insane person is absorbed in his or her own fan-
tasies that no one else perceives.

All these are not merely aberrations in the brain. They
may include psychic abilities or psychic sensitivities but
are beyond the control of the person. The person may connect up to the astral plane and lose contact with physical
realities. In these cases, the mind goes into an absorption
of the dull or blank type and sometimes an astral entity
comes in to use the mind. All severe mental derangement
involves such possessions by influences or entities, in
which we lose conscious control of the mind.[85]

Spiritual and Non-spiritual Samadhis

There can be a combination of higher and lower Samadhis. These include powerful or enduring mystical experiences that are mixed with egoism. The person has a legit-
imate deep experience but the ego colors it. We feel that
we are the avatar, Jesus Christ or some other great holy
person, or that God is giving a special revelation through
us. Some of the religious cults that have caused trouble in
the world are based upon such mystical experiences which
were authentic but of a mixed nature. Being exposed to a

person in such a mixed Samadhi can be very deranging, particularly for the naive or the unprepared. The authenticity of their Samadhi causes one to believe their ego delusions.

Lower Samadhis are externally directed and based upon desire. The higher Samadhis are produced by the mind itself when it transcends desire. Some intermediate Samadhis exist in that there is desire but of a more subtle nature, such as can be experienced in astral travel, in which we may find subtle forms of enjoyment in worlds beyond the physical. These also come under the Samadhis of the one-pointed mind but can be mixed in nature.

Samadhi and Prana

Samadhi of some kind occurs whenever the mind becomes fully absorbed in Prana or vital energy and its functions. Our vital functions draw and hold the mind. Moreover, extra Prana is required to sustain the mind, which is very mobile, in any condition of absorption. If we do not have the energy to focus the mind, it will wander off. In Samadhi, the mind itself gets absorbed in the Prana or the energy of an experience, which leaves a powerful imprint on the psyche. Only those powerful experiences which are invested with a great deal of Prana can hold the mind. In this regard Prana is also of three types — Sattvic, Rajasic and Tamasic.

Tamasic Prana operates in states of sleep, stupor, coma, or under the influence of drugs — the Samadhis of the deluded mind. The mind gets absorbed in this Tamasic Prana and feels calm. However one's problems have not been solved but merely covered over by ignorance.

Rajasic Prana operates during motor activities, like eating, drinking, eliminating, having sex, or during any state of strong exertion like running or working, and during sensory activities that are overwhelming, like experiences of great pleasure, pain, joy, sorrow, fear or attachment. These are the Samadhis of the disturbed mind.

Pranic experiences in general are dominated by Rajas and so all powerful Pranic activities have an effect on the level of the Rajasic mind. Any vital (Pranic) function involves at least a temporary absorption of the mind, even eating or defecating. The active Prana holds the mind for the purpose of discharging its function without interference from other activities. The mind is suspended until Prana achieves the aim of its action. Whenever Prana performs a vital function, the mind must be put in abeyance during the time that function is discharged, even if it is only an instance. Whenever Prana acts, the mind gets absorbed to some degree. Observe how your mind internalizes, at least a little, during eating or any other vital action.

Sattvic Prana operates during states of inspiration like artistic inspiration, genius, and any sort of creative insight or invention from the scientific to the philosophical. This feeling of inspiration is itself a form of Prana. It results from investing our life energy in some creative work. To some extent, Samadhi of a Sattvic Prana occurs during all our sensory perceptions, particularly seeing and hearing, because the mind must be temporarily absorbed in a Sattvic state of illumination for perception to occur. These sensory Samadhis, however, endure only for an instant and so are missed unless the mind is already very subtle and pure.

Yogic Samadhis similarly require a special energization of the Prana to achieve them and occur when the mind and Prana are united consciously. For this reason Pranayama is very important in creating yogic Samadhis. Without developing an increased energy of Prana, it is very difficult to reach these yogic Samadhis. Prana and Chitta, the vital force and our deeper consciousness, are connected, as we have already noted in our discussion of Chitta. One should not forget the role of Prana in Samadhi, either of a higher or lower nature.

Psychoanalysis often fails because it does not get to the level of Prana and Chitta — the subconscious mind in which our mental afflictions are lodged — and the Prana that these hold. Releasing the Prana behind our psychological states is not an intellectual exercise. One of the best ways to do this is to practice Pranayama. As one does Pranayama, the subconscious gets energized and deep-seated patterns come up. If one consciously breathes deeply through these emotional afflictions, they automatically get released, even if one does not examine the outer circumstances that originally brought them about. In this way Prana can be used to clear our deeper consciousness and lead us into higher states of absorption.

Samadhi and Ayurvedic Psychology

Ayurvedic psychology examines the lower or illusory Samadhis and employs its methods, from diet to meditation, to help remove their conditioning upon the mind. As states of Samadhi, their impact on the psyche can be very great and hard to remove. The general rule is: Only if a higher Samadhi is developed can the effects of a lower Samadhi be completely neutralized. In fact, all true spiritual practices develop higher (spiritual) Samadhis to counter the lower (worldly) Samadhis and their attachments.

Yogic practices develop a higher form of Samskara (mental tendency) using postures, breathing exercises, mantra and meditation to create a state of consciousness based upon love, peace and wisdom. Only a higher or Sattvic Samskara can counter the effects of lower, Rajasic and Tamasic, Samskaras. This alone can counter our ordinary tendencies with their imprint of lesser Samadhis based upon desire, disturbance and illusion. Once these higher Samskaras are developed, they lead us to the spiritual life in which we can transcend even them to a state of pure awareness.

Lesser mental disorders usually involve attachment to a lesser Samadhi, like addictions to sex, alcohol, or food. Until the person learns a higher type of absorption, the Samskaras of these lesser Samadhis will draw the mind back to them and recreate their behavior. However, it is not always possible to take people from the lesser to the higher Samadhis. Sometimes it is necessary to proceed by stages, developing Samadhis of the distracted mind to counter those of the deluded mind and then Samadhis of the imaginative mind to counter those of the deluded mind.

Some of the lower Samadhis of the imaginative or distracted mind can be useful in treatment. If an emotionally disturbed person can develop absorption in some useful activity, this can help calm the mind. Getting patients to take up some active physical exercise program (developing a Samadhi of the distracted mind), and getting into the joy of it, can help counter psychological problems. Similarly, getting them interested in artistic expression (Samadhis of the imaginative mind) can help them yet further.

To help a psychologically disturbed person discover more wholesome Samadhis is the key to treatment. This is the purpose of Ayurvedic psychological therapies, particularly subtle sensory therapies, mantra and meditation. We

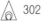

must learn the appropriate places to allow our minds to be absorbed. These should be Sattvic influences or the mind will remain ignorant and disturbed. We must learn to develop the higher Samadhis so that we are not trapped in the lower. We must learn to develop internal states of absorption that are enduring, or our minds must remain trapped in external absorptions and the pain of their coming to an end.

Summary of the Eightfold Yogic Path

The eight limbs of Yoga reflect the process by which our minds work, which has to be oriented the right way for peace of mind.

1. First, we have certain values of social conduct that determine how we relate to the world (Yamas). Most important is the violence we allow in our lives (ahimsa), how truthful we are, how we use our sexual energy, what possessions we keep around us, and what we are most deeply attached to. These create our psychological atmosphere.

2. Second, closely related to these are the rules of our personal conduct and lifestyle (Niyamas). We have a certain way of acting in which we find our main contentment. We organize our outer life in a certain manner. We have a certain way of looking at ourselves and who we are. We follow a certain discipline or routine. We have a particular way of seeking help or favor from others. This determines how we live.

For example, if you want to make money, you must

place your seeking of happiness in that goal. You must organize your outer life accordingly, eliminating those things that inhibit the achievement of wealth. This gives you a certain identity or sense of self. It creates a discipline, like work in the business world. You must also gain the help of those who can grant what you seek, like those in positions of power.

Whatever we decide to do, even if it is the pursuit of pleasure, creates certain values and disciplines. We must give up one thing in order to gain another. Life always involves choice and action always involves some methodology to achieve the goals we choose.

This basic lifestyle orientation underlies our psychology. Wrong values and wrong practices that arise from them cause psychological disorders. Sometimes the value is wrong, like seeking to harm others. Sometimes the approach is wrong, like seeking love but in ways that bring us into contact with people who exploit us. Wrong life-orientation causes the mind to open itself up to factors of disturbance and sorrow. Yet whatever type of action we pursue requires some basic orientation of our energies, from taking a trip to planning a career.

3. Third, based on our orientation in life, we have a way of movement that holds the body in a particular posture. The pursuit of sexual pleasure causes us to use the body in one way, the pursuit of athletic excellence is another, and so on. Certain ways of orienting the body increase stress and tension, cause debility or disease, or in other ways contribute to psychological distress.

4. Fourth, we have a specific way of using our vital energy (Pranayama). Whatever we decide to do directs our Prana toward that particular goal. Whatever we do, we are investing that action with our vitality, which in turn molds our vitality. If we are pursuing art, sports, business or spirituality, each will cause a particular orientation of the vital force.

5. Fifth, we have a way of focusing our mind and senses (Pratyahara). At any given moment there are innumerable sensory impressions coming into the mind and we must select a few to consider based upon the choices we have made in our behavior. Whether it is watching television, working at our office desk, or just walking down the street, we are withdrawing from certain sensations in order to focus on others. If the sensations we are focusing on are unwholesome (Rajasic and Tamasic), then the mind must be distorted in the process.

6. Sixth, we must direct our attention in a specific direction (Dharana). What we choose to do in life creates a certain focus of attention. It not only eliminates other objects from our attention but concentrates us on the chosen object. If that object or goal is unwholesome, our mental energy will be concentrated in a painful way.

7. Seventh, we have certain things that we reflect upon deeply (Dhyana) — the most constant objects of our thoughts. We are always thinking about something. Our thoughts circulate around the goals we are seeking, our basic enjoyments, acquisitions and achievements. If the main

objects that we reflect upon are disturbing, limited or confused, then the mental field must be distorted as well.

8. Eighth, we must absorb our minds in those things we most seek. This will occur in certain peak experiences (Samadhi) that come at the end of our striving. Even the attainment of pleasurable objects, like sex or food, is the culmination of certain values and disciplines and seldom comes without effort. The same is true for other goals of life. However, if the object we seek is tinged with personal craving, our absorption in it must be transient and leaves us feeling empty, however happy that moment of absorption may be.

Yoga is a way of doing this process consciously, in which we gain absorption in God or our true nature. Psychological disorders occur through doing it wrongly or unconsciously, in which we gain absorption in wrong influences that cause us to lose power over our own consciousness (lose our inner peace). Once we understand this process, we will no longer seek those things that bring us suffering. This requires truly understanding our consciousness and how it works. Without understanding and applying the great principles of Yoga and Ayurveda, we cannot do this.

May you, the reader, proceed quickly and without hindrance on this great path of immortal life!

Primary Yantra

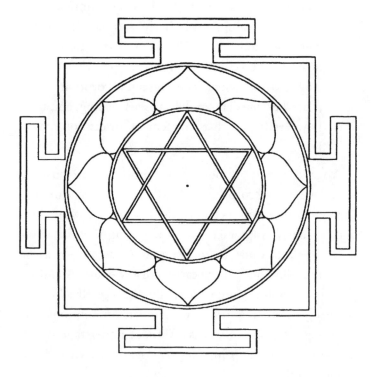

Appendix 1

The following tables provide not only a summary but a more extensive knowledge of our psycho-physical nature and its place in the greater universe of consciousness. Topics covered are the three bodies, the five sheaths, the seven levels of the universe, the seven chakras, the five Pranas, a table of the functions of the mind (Chitta), and a diagram of cosmic evolution.

Table A
The Three Bodies

Our true Self, whose nature is Pure Consciousness, is encased in three bodies or vestures. Only the gross or physical body is a body in the ordinary sense of the word. The subtle (astral) body is built up from the impressions derived through the mind and senses. The causal body is made up of our most deep-seated tendencies, held in the three gunas of sattva, rajas and tamas. The inner Self is the fourth factor that transcends the three bodies.

Body	Composition	State	Existence	Guna
Gross (Physical)	gross elements derived from food	waking	physical	tamas
Subtle (Astral)	subtle elements derived from impressions	dream	astral	rajas
Causal	causal elements derived from gunas	deep sleep	causal or ideal	sattva
Transcendent beyond Self (Pure Consciousness)	unmodified consciousness	transcendent (turiya)	unmanifest absolute	gunas

The physical body functions during the waking state, in which we live in a world of physical objects, each with its specific form and location in time and space. For this body to exist, we must eat and take in the gross elements that compose it.

The astral body functions during dream and inspired thought, in which we live in the world of our own impressions. It defines time and space rather than being defined by them. It is sustained by impressions and the subtle elements, which are its food. It is dominated by the emotional or sense-mind (Manas).

The causal body functions during deep sleep and profound meditation, in which we live in our own consciousness devoid of external objects, perceived or imaginary. It is not located as a form or impression in space and time, but exists as an idea that creates time and space according to its qualities. It is sustained by thoughts, the causal elements, which are its food. It is dominated by our deeper consciousness (Chitta). Our true Self and immortal being transcend all three bodies and states of consciousness. Only in this rests our liberation from time and space, birth and death.

The Three Bodies and Psychological Disorders

We must determine the level of our nature from which our psychological problems derive in order to treat them properly. If their cause is physical, like wrong diet, it must be treated on that level. If the cause is astral, like wrong impressions, these impressions must be changed to improve the condition. If the cause is causal, like deep-seated rajas and tamas in the soul, they are difficult to correct and their causes may stem from past life karma. Treating them physically and astrally improves them indirectly.

It is difficult to get to the causal level directly because this requires control of the lower bodies and the ability to meditate.

Physical disease factors, like bad food or water, affect the astral body indirectly according to the impressions derived from them. In the same way, impressions in the astral body affect the causal body indirectly according to their gunas. All three bodies are involved in some way, whatever the condition is.

Relative to healing, our physical world can be changed by altering the objects around which we live, and particularly those we ingest (food, water and air). Our astral world can be changed by altering our impressions and ideas. Our causal world can be changed by altering our deepest beliefs and desires (the gunas we hold to).

Table B
The Five Sheaths and the Mind

The three bodies make up five sheaths or layers of matter from the gross physical to the causal.

Layer	Sheath	Function	Composition
Chitta (Consciousness or inner mind)	Bliss, Anandamaya Kosha	love or spiritual aspiration	Samskaras (Guna imprints from tanmatras)
Buddhi (Intelligence) tis)	intelligence, Vijnanamaya kosha	reason or discernment	mental activities (Vrit-
Manas (Outer mind)	sensory, Manomaya kosha	gathering sensory and data	impressions (tanmatras)
Prana (Vital force)	vital, Pranamaya kosha	animate the physical and astral bodies	five Pranas
Physical	food, Annamaya kosha	allow for embodiment	five Elements

The three bodies constitute five sheaths. The Pranic sheath mediates between the physical and astral bodies; the intelligence sheath mediates between the astral and causal. The three main functions of the mind (Chitta, Buddhi and Manas) constitute the three most subtle sheaths. The field of our core-consciousness makes up the sheath of bliss (Anandamaya Kosha) in which we hold our deeper joys and sorrows, our karmas and Samskaras that are imprinted in the gunas. Consciousness is bliss, with love or desire being predominant, ever seeking happiness and joy. It governs the state of deep sleep in which all manifest thoughts and impressions disappear and in which we experience peace and joy.

The field of intelligence makes up the sheath of intelligence, in which we hold our deeper knowledge, judgments and discrimination of truth. This either allows us access to the bliss sheath, if our wisdom is spiritual, or closes it off to us, if our knowledge is of the outer world only. This is the site of most of our mental activities (vrittis), particularly those that relate to the determination of truth and reality.

The field of the mind makes up the mental sheath, in which we hold our various impressions, both sensory and mental. These either allow us access to the intelligence sheath, if we have understood and digested them, or close it off, if we are caught in outer enjoyments.

Pranamaya kosha's lower (Tamasic) aspect becomes the physical Pranas, its higher (Rajasic) aspect becomes the subtle Pranas and emotions (mind and senses) and constitutes the emotional body. Similarly, the intelligence sheath is dual in nature. Its lower (Rajasic) function is intellect, or thought directed toward the outer world, which works along with the senses and part of the astral body. Its higher (Sattvic) function is true intelligence, or discrimination directed toward the eternal part of the causal body, and transcends the senses.

TABLE C
THE SEVEN LEVELS OF THE UNIVERSE

The universe is an organic entity or Cosmic Person constructed by Cosmic Intelligence and occurring in different layers — from Pure Being to gross physical matter. The five sheaths correspond to the first five levels of the universe.

1. MATTER ....Anna
2. ENERGY........................Prana
3. EMOTION ....Manas
4. INTELLIGENCE ....Vijnana
5. BLISS ....Ananda
6. CONSCIOUSNESS ....Chit
7. BEING............................Sat

Being and Consciousness, the last two, have no sheaths because they are beyond all manifestation. They are the fundamental reality and background of the other principles, which can be viewed as a series of concentric circles with the physical in the middle as the most limited factor. They create seven worlds, lokas or planes of existence.

Ananda, Bliss, is dual in nature, with its higher aspect beyond manifestation and its lower aspect being the source of manifestation. Together with the other higher two principles, it forms Sacchidananda, Being-Consciousness-Bliss, as the threefold transcendent reality of Brahman or Atman, the Absolute or Self.

TABLE D
THE SEVEN CHAKRAS

The Chakras are energy fields in the subtle body and govern the subtle elements, sense organs, and organs of action. They possess corresponding energy fields in the physical body, the nerve plexus, which similarly govern gross elements, the physical sense organs and organs of action. A tendency of New Age thought is to confuse the outer or physical function of the chakras with their inner or spiritual function, which is quite different and only comes into play during advanced meditation practices.

Element	Location	Sense Quality	Sense Organ	Motor Organ
Consciousness	Head	Causal Sound	Causal Hearing and Speech	
Mind	Third Eye	Subtle Sound	Subtle Hearing and Speech	
Ether	Throat	Sound	Ears	Vocal Organ
Air	Heart	Touch	Skin	Hands
Fire	Navel	Sight	Eyes	Feet
Water	Sex	Taste	Tongue	Reproductive Organs
Earth	Root	Smell	Nose	Organs of Elimination

Derangement in the mind gets reflected by disharmonies in the respective chakras and their functions, along with the inability of the higher chakra functions to come into play. The five lower chakras in their outer function relate to the physical sensory and motor organs. In their heightened or spiritual function, they awaken the subtle sensory and motor organs to which they relate, giving us the experience of subtle worlds and higher states of consciousness.

Psychological problems relate to their respective chakras and depress their function. Lack of control of the sense organs prevents their respective chakras from opening and keeps their function weak or deranged. For example, excess sexual activity weakens the water chakra and prevents it from opening, while excess fear damages the earth chakra. Control of the senses brings the energy of consciousness inward for the unfoldment of its higher aspects. The role of the third eye is crucial in this regard because through it the senses are concentrated and directed within.

Ayurvedic psychology balances Vata, Pitta and Kapha in the body and increases Sattva in the mind to harmonize lower chakra functions and creates the foundation for the opening of their higher potential. Tejas helps open the lower chakras and corresponds to Kundalini. Ojas aids in the unfoldment of the higher chakras of the head and third eye. Prana allows the heart (air) chakra to open. Control of Manas gives us control of the lower five chakras. Development of Buddhi allows the third eye to develop. Clearing of the Chitta opens the crown chakra and the deeper spiritual heart. Dissolution of the ego (Ahamkara) is the key to the process because ego creates the constriction of energy that prevents the chakras from functioning properly.

TABLE E
THE FIVE PRANAS AND THE MIND

Prana is divided fivefold according to its movement and function.

Prana	physical location	physical function	subtle function
Vyana Vayu— diffusive vital force	heart and limbs, pervades entire body	movement and circulation	mental circulation and expansion
Udana Vayu— ascending vital force	throat, upper chest	speech, exhalation, growth	aspiration, enthusiasm, effort, mental growth
Prana Vayu— tion inward moving vital force	heart and brain	swallowing, inhalation, sensory perception	mental energiza- and receptivity
Samana Vayu— equalizing vital force	navel	digestion and metabolism, homeostasis	mental digestion and homeostasis
Apana Vayu— downward moving vital force	below the navel	elimination, reproduction, immunity	mental elimination and immunity

These five Pranas are all diversifications of the air element, its subtle counterpart (the tanmatra or sensory quality of touch), and the guna of Rajas. The five Pranas are common to all the elements, organs, koshas, and functions of the mind. They serve to energize and to connect our activities on all levels.

Prana brings about energization. Samana provides nutrition. Apana is responsible for elimination. Vyana governs circulation. Udana provides for effort and the capacity to work. For example, on the physical level, Prana is responsible for eating food, Samana for digesting it, Vyana circulates the nutrients to all the tissues, Apana eliminates the waste material from the food, and Udana allows us to use the energy derived from the food for physical work.

On the level of the mind, Prana is responsible for the intake of impressions and ideas, Samana digests them, Vyana circulates this information, Apana removes the waste material (negative thoughts and emotions), and Udana allows us to do positive mental work and exertion.

On a general level, Prana energizes all the koshas, Samana sustains their relationship, cohesion and balance, Apana brings energy down the koshas from the subtle to the gross, Udana brings energy up the koshas from the gross to the subtle, and Vyana brings about circulation through all the five koshas and is responsible for their differentiation.

Psychological Disorders and the Pranas

Psychological disorders involve imbalances in the Pranas or energies that govern the mind. First, Prana or energization is disturbed by taking in wrong impressions, emotions or thoughts. Second, Samana or digestion gets imbalanced through wrong intakes and poor discrimination. Then the other three Pranas become disturbed. Apana brings about the increase of waste materials in the mind. Vyana or circulation is impaired, bringing about stagnation in our deeper consciousness. Udana or our positive will is weakened and we are unable to make the efforts to change or improve our condition.

Prana Vayu is our ability to absorb positive impressions and thoughts, as well as the capacity of the life-force to control our equilibrium. Disturbed, it prevents us from bringing in positive impressions and sets our entire equilibrium off balance. This guiding Prana is connected with

Agni or the fire principle and together with it vitalizes the mind and senses.

Apana Vayu is our ability to ward off negativity, the force of gravity in the mind. When its function is deranged, we get depressed or take in the energies of stagnation and decay. Various disturbed downward flows of the life-energy can occur.

Samana Vayu, the equalizing life-energy, is weakened when mental peace and harmony are disturbed. Physically, this deranges the digestive system and weakens absorption, allowing for the build-up of toxins. This causes psychological congestion and attachment, along with the inability to be alone. Severe psychological problems may cause significant Samana Vayu disorders, with derangement of the nervous system and long-term mental imbalance.

Vyana Vayu is the expansive part of the life-energy, responsible for outward-directed movement and activity. It makes us happy, independent and expansive. Disturbed, it causes tremors in the body or agitation in the mind. In the mind, it causes alienation and isolation and prevents us from getting along with other people.

Udana Vayu is our ascending enthusiasm, will and motivation. It makes us feel elated, proud or exalted. It gets weakened by depression. When we are depressed, our energy is unable to move upwards and sinks. Inability to speak or express ourselves indicates that Udana Vayu is weak. Various disturbed upward flows of the life-force can occur, like coughing or uncontrolled speech when this Prana is deranged. In excess, it makes us vain, domineering and intolerant.

These five Pranas are one of the most profound aspects of Ayurvedic thought. We are only introducing them here, but their role should not be underestimated. They require a book on them alone.

TABLE F
FUNCTIONS OF THE MIND

Self or Soul ....**Jivatman**
Element..........................Ether aspect of Subtle Air and Ether
....Elements
Guna ....Unmanifest condition of Gunas
Sheath ....Bliss Sheath fully activated
Functions ....Self-awareness
Sense ....Self-realization
State of Awareness ....Ever-waking
State of Time ....Eternal Present
Kingdom of Nature ......Yogi or Sage
Nature ....Pure Knowledge

Consciousness ....**Chitta**
Element ....Air aspect of Subtle Air and Ether
Guna ....Source of the Gunas
Sheath ....Bliss Sheath in general
Functions ....Memory, Sleep, Samadhi
Sense ....Instinct/Intuition
State of Time ....Past
State of Awareness ....Deep Sleep
Kingdom of Nature ......Plant (lower), God or angel (higher)
Nature ....Love, Desire

Intelligence ....**Buddhi**
Element ....Fire aspect of Subtle Air and Ether
Guna ....Sattva
Sheath ....Intelligence Sheath
Functions ....Perception, Reason, Determination
Sense ....Sense Organs, particularly hearing

State of Time..................Present
State of Awareness ....Waking
Kingdom of Nature........Human (Sage when fully activated)
Nature............................Knowledge, Higher and Lower

Mind...........................Manas
Element..........................Water aspect of Subtle Air and Ether
Guna ....Rajas
Sheath ....Mind Sheath
Functions ....Sensation, Volition, Imagination
Sense- ....Organs of Action, particularly hands
State of Time..................Future
State of Awareness..........Dream
Kingdom of Nature ......Animal
Nature ....Action

Ego ....Ahamkara
Element..........................Earth aspect of Subtle Air and Ether
Guna ....Tamas
Sheath ....Physical body
Functions ....Self-sense, ownership
Sense ....Self or ego
State of Time..................Past
State of Awareness ....Deep sleep
Kingdom of Nature ......Elemental
Nature............................Ignorance

Appendix 2

Footnotes

1 This is called Yoga-chikitsa in Sanskrit. Yoga as spiritual practice is called Yoga-sadhana.

2 Similarly, classical yogic texts employ Ayurvedic terminology to describe the physiological effects of yogic practices.

3 Ayurveda like Yoga is based upon the Sankhya philosophy which derives from the Upanishads.

4 This follows the attributions of the elements and the sensory capacities that we note later in the book.

5 For more information on Prana, Tejas and Ojas, note my book TANTRIC YOGA AND THE WISDOM GODDESSES: Spiritual Secrets of Ayurveda, pages 193-226. It includes the signs and conditions of high, low or sufficient Prana, Tejas and Ojas. It has a section on how to develop them and how to keep them in balance.

6 For a more traditional but more complex examination of sattvic, rajasic and tamasic mental types in Ayurveda, note CHARAKA SAMHITA, SARIRASTHANA IV. 36-40.

7 Psychiatry with its use of chemical drugs can be a Tamasic therapy. It is mainly useful in cases of excess Rajas in which the patient can cause harm to himself or others. Drugs can be useful short term in other high Rajasic conditions like acute pain or severe anxiety, which may require strong sedation. As drugs are Tamasic in nature, their long term effect is to inhibit Sattva. They must be used only as a last resort or temporary measure.

8 Psychoanalysis is generally a Rajasic therapy. It takes us from repressed emotions (Tamas) to self-expression (rajas). However, it may not lead us to Sattva unless additional therapies are added. Analysis must lead to practical action. Excess analysis can prevent a person from really changing, just as thinking about a problem too much can prevent us from dealing with it.

9 Modern psychoanalysis, with its active and communicative methods, is essentially a Rajasic process. It aims at breaking up and releasing repressed (Tamasic) emotional patterns. Analysis helps bring the mind from a Tamasic (repressed) to a Rajasic

(thoughtful, active and motivated) state.

10   What is called karma yoga in Sanskrit.

11   This witnessing attitude is called Sakshi-bhava in Sanskrit and
     is the basis of most Vedantic forms of meditation.

12   This is the Atman of Vedantic thought.

13   According to the YOGA SUTRAS III.33, meditation upon the
     heart brings knowledge of the mind.

14   Note Patanjali, YOGA SUTRA I.2. "Yoga is the mastery of all
     the operations of consciousness (Chitta)."

15   In the Buddhist Yogachara school, this deeper consciousness is
     called Alaya Vijnana or "storehouse consciousness" for its retain-
     ing all karmic tendencies.

16   Unconditioned Chit reflected into matter (Prakriti or Maya)
     becomes conditioned chitta. However, we should note that in
     Buddhist teachings, like the Lankavatara Sutra, the term chitta
     can refer to conditioned chitta or unconditioned Chit. The latter
     is called unconditioned chitta or the pure nature of Mind. The
     One Mind of Buddhism, Eka Chitta, referring to the uncondi-
     tioned One Consciousness, resembles the One Self or Atman, of
     Vedantic thought.

17   Iccha predominant in Sanskrit.

18   Ayurveda discusses the importance of truthful memory in detail
     in CHARAKA SAMHITA, SARIRASTHANA I.147-151, as a
     means of both health and liberation.

19   Note section on Samadhi in Yoga chapter of the book for more
     information.

20   Ayurveda discusses the role of wrong use of intelligence under
     the term Prajnaparadha or failure of wisdom. Note CARAKA
     SAMHITA, SARIRASTHANA I.102-109.

21   The BHAGAVAD GITA, the great yogic scripture of the avatar
     Krishna, emphasizes Buddhi Yoga, the Yoga of Intelligence,
     through which we can maintain equanimity throughout all the
     ups and downs of life.

22   This is called viveka in Sanskrit.

23   This Cosmic Intelligence is called Mahat in Sanskrit. It is the
     cosmic counterpart of Buddhi.

24   These are called Brahma, Vishnu and Shiva in Hindu thought.

25 This is the higher aspect of Agni or the Cosmic Fire.

26 Sanskrit antarayami.

27 Compared to consciousness (Chitta) in its original form, even the higher aspect of intelligence appears Rajasic. For this reason, some yogis relate Chitta to Sattva and Buddhi to Rajas. Other times, however, Chitta and Buddhi are identified because both are predominantly Sattvic, which is the view of Classical Samkhya. In the same way, Cosmic Intelligence and Cosmic Consciousness are often regarded as the same.

28 For this reason it is also sometimes located in the throat, or between the head and the heart.

29 Jnana predominant in Sanskrit.

30 This is called Prajnaparadha in Sanskrit and is one the main causative factors in the disease process according to Ayurveda.

31 This will to truth is called Kratu in the Vedas, which implies sacrifice or self-negation. This only comes through intelligence which negates our outer desires. It requires the alignment of intelligence and the mind, in which the mind's desires are directed inward through renunciation. Later Vedanta calls it Samkalpa Shakti or true will power, doing what we say and saying what we do.

32 The section on Samadhi in the chapter on consciousness is also relevant here.

33 This immersion of intelligence (Buddhi) in the heart (Chitta) is called Bodhichitta or enlightened consciousness in Buddhist thought.

34 Manas occurs as a general term for the mind in Vedantic literature, in which case it is synonymous with chitta and includes all the other functions of the mind under its scope. In Buddhist literature, Manas can refer to all the functions of the mind. The unconditioned Manas can refer to the Buddha nature or enlightened awareness, like the Atman of Vedanta. As most mental activity occurs in the field of Manas, it can be considered as the most characteristic part of what we normally call the mind.

35 Actors learn to play with these core feelings or emotions. They are called rasas or essences in Sanskrit. They are also referred to as bhavas, or states of feeling, which in turn reflect various relationships. Feeling is relationship-oriented. To work with these feelings and relationships consciously is the path of devotion,

Bhakti Yoga.

36 Some Yogis classify Manas as tamas compared to Buddhi as Satt-
    va because Manas has an outgoing and Buddhi an ingoing ener-
    gy. Manas does have a component of Tamas, and Rajas generally
    leads to Tamas. Classical Samkhya makes Manas a product of
    Ahamkara or ego, deriving it from its Sattvic and Rajasic sides.
    This reflects the relationship between Manas and the sensory
    and motor organs, which are related to Sattva and Rajas respec-
    tively. All the functions of the mind need some Sattva in order
    to function clearly.

37 Sanskrit kriya.

38 Vata people, however, have the most active and generally most
    disturbed minds. This is because they are most sensitive and
    because their consciousness (Chitta) is most exposed through the
    actions of both body and mind.

39 Sanskrit samkalpa and vikalpa. Yet here it is ordinary samkalpa,
    or intention to action, with the body and senses, not the higher
    will or samkalpa, the will to truth, which requires alignment
    with the Buddhi and the Self.

40 This is called Samkalpa Shakti in Sanskrit, the power of will or
    intention. Cultivating it means that we set spiritual goals for
    ourselves, like controlling our anger, and then accomplish these,
    whatever the effort it may take.

41 This is called Aham-dhi or Aham-buddhi in Sanskrit, showing
    that it is a mistake or misconception of intelligence or Buddhi.

42 This has been a Vedantic criticism of certain Buddhist systems.

43 These are called ahamtva and mamatva in Sanskrit.

44 These two factors are discussed in the chapter on Spiritual
    Methods of Treatment.

45 Ayurvedic literature contains extensive discussions of the indi-
    vidual soul and Supreme Soul and their relationship. Note
    CARAKA SAMHITA, SARIRASTHANA I.

46 Note particularly the teachings of the modern teacher Ramana
    Maharshi and the ancient teacher Shankara for the teachings of
    Advaita or non-dualistic Vedanta. Other Vedantic approaches
    exist as well, like the integral non-dualism (Purnadvaita) of Sri
    Aurobindo, the qualified non-dualism (Visishtadvaita) of
    Ramanuja, and the dualistic Vedanta of Madhva.

47 Chitta-shuddhi in Sanskrit.

48 In ordinary Ayurvedic terminology, the Doshas of Vata, Pitta and Kapha in excess damage the tissues or dhatus of the body, which is the dushti or damaged factor. In Ayurvedic psychology, Buddhi-dosha causes Chitta-dushti, wrong functioning of intelligence damages the substance of our consciousness.

49 For an extensive examination of these different functions of the mind and their states according to the three gunas note SCIENCE OF THE SOUL by Swami Yogeshwaranand Saraswati, pages 96-115.

50 Note YOGA SUTRAS II. 33-34.

51 Please examine the section on intelligence for more information on the right function of the Buddhi.

52 These three states relate to Vaishvanara, Taijasa and Prajna in Vedantic thought. Vaishvanara is the digestive fire in the physical body. Taijasa is the digestive fire in the subtle body. Prajna is the digestive fire in the causal body. Taijasa, the power of Tejas, being the digestive fire in the subtle body or mind is most important in the digestion of impressions or mental digestion.

53 Note section on Pancha Karma later in the book, pages 202-203

54 Note CARAKA SAMHITA, SARIRASTHANA I.118-132 for an examination of the role of the senses in the disease process.

55 For example, my book AYURVEDIC HEALING, pages 51-87, in this regard.

56 Unfortunately there are many animal additives to foods, like fish liver oil as a vitamin supplement, rennet in cheese, or cows' bones used to bleach sugar. One should try to avoid these as well.

57 This has been outlined in AYURVEDIC HEALING, pages 83-85.

58 Note YOGA OF HERBS in this regard.

59 For a materia medica of the herbs mentioned in this book, please consult YOGA OF HERBS and PLANETARY HERBOLOGY.

60 Note YOGA OF HERBS, pages 23-25, for its discussion of the six tastes.

61 These are called medhya rasayanas in Sanskrit.

62   These five practices are called vamana, virechana, basti, nasya and raktamoksha in Sanskrit.

63   Note CARAKA SAMHITA, SUTRASTHANA XI.54 where gems are listed among the spiritual therapies of Ayurveda.

64   More information on Vedic astrology, including its healing aspects, is presented in ASTROLOGY OF THE SEERS, particularly pages 235-261.

65   For more information on the Ayurvedic use of gems, examine AYURVEDIC HEALING, pages 308-312.

66   Note CARAKA SAMHITA SUTRASTHANA XI.54 where mantra is mentioned among the spiritual therapies of Ayurveda.

67   This process is called purascharana or anusthana in Sanskrit.

68   This subject is examined in TANTRIC YOGA AND THE WISDOM GODDESSES. Also look into Haresh Johari's TOOLS FOR TANTRA.

69   Note TANTRIC YOGA AND THE WISDOM GODDESSES, pages 197-219, for ways of increasing Prana, Tejas and Ojas, including mantra.

70   This chosen form of God is called Ishta Devata in Sanskrit. There are many works on Bhakti Yoga or the Yoga of Devotion, like the BHAKTI SUTRAS of Narada, SRIMAD BHAGA-VATAM, the RAMAYANA, and the songs of great saints like Mira Bai.

71   These are called homa, havana and Agnihotra in Sanskrit.

72   In TANTRIC YOGA AND THE WISDOM GODDESSES, I examined the role of ten important Goddesses in this regard.

73   Vagbhatta, the great Buddhist Ayurvedic teacher, recommended using the Bodhisattva Avalokiteshvara or the Gods Shiva and Vishnu (ASTANGAHRDAYA UTTARASTHANA V.50-52). Avalokiteshvara's consort is the Goddess Tara, also called Kwan Yin in the Chinese tradition.

74   Self-knowledge is the subject matter of Advaita or non-dualistic Vedanta. Its main classical proponent is Shankaracharya. Its most noted modern proponent is Ramana Maharshi, the great sage of Tiruvannamalai, South India.

75   For the importance of Yoga in traditional Ayurveda, note CARAKA SAMHITA, SARIRASTHANA I.137- 155.

76 YOGA SUTRAS of Patanjali, Book I, Sutra 2.

77 What are called varna and ashrama in Vedic thought. The var-
nas are our social ethic, which is divided into four as it is based
on knowledge, honor, wealth or work. The ashramas are the
stages of life as youth, householder, retiree and renunciate.

78 The true purpose of Yoga is inner integration. It is done for a
spiritual purpose and requires renunciation and self-abnegation.
Enjoyment, called bhoga in Sanskrit, is not the aim of Yoga,
which moves in another direction. However, many people do
Yoga in order to feel better, which is a pursuit of bhoga. This
often distorts what Yoga means and prevents us from benefiting
from its deeper practices.

79 Note YOGA SUTRAS I.12. Vyasa's commentary, for an explanation of Chitta-Nadi. The outer flow of the mind through the
senses leads to bondage and sorrow. The inner flow through discrimination leads to peace and liberation. this inner flow sets in
motion the Kundalini, which is the awakened Chitta-Nadi.

80 This is called Shambahvi mudra in yogic thought. It is used in
several systems of Buddhist meditation as well.

81 We have already discussed Samadhi in the sections of the book
on Chitta and Buddhi and will not repeat that information here.
Please keep it in mind.

82 Vyasa, the main commentator on YOGA SUTRAS, defines
Yoga as Samadhi. The first section of the book is the Samadhi
Pada or section relating to Samadhi. The majority of verses in
the book relate to Samadhi or Samyama.

83 Sanskrit — note Vyasa's commentary on first verse of YOGA
SUTRAS.

84 These Samadhis (samyamas) are explained in great detail in the
YOGA SUTRAS, particularly the third section.

85 These types of possession are explained in Ayurvedic psychology.
I have examined some of these in AYURVEDIC HEALING,
pages 254-257.

Sanskrit Glossary

Agni - digestive fire,

Ahamkara - ego or sense of separate self

Antahkarana - internal instrument, mind on all levels

Apana - downward moving Prana

Asanas - yogic postures

Astral Plane - subtle world of pure impressions, dream plane

Atman - true Self, sense of pure I am

Ayurveda - yogic science of healing

Bhakti Yoga - Yoga of Devotion

Bija Mantra - single syllable mantras like OM

Brahman - Absolute reality

Buddhi - intelligence

Causal Plane - source world of creation, realm of the ideal or archetypes, deep sleep plane

Chakras - energy centers of subtle body, which govern the physical body through the nerve plexus

Chitta - consciousness, inner mind, particularly the subconscious

Devi - the Goddess

Dharana - concentration

Dharma - the law of our nature

Dhyana - meditation

Gunas - three prime qualities of Nature of sattva, rajas and tamas

Guru - spiritual guide

Homa - Vedic fire offerings

Ishvara - God or the Creator

Ishvari - Divine Mother, feminine aspect of God

Jiva - individual soul

Jnana Yoga - Yoga of Self-knowledge

Karma - effect of our past actions, including from
    previous births

Karma Yoga - yoga of ritual, work and service

Kundalini - latent energy of spiritual development

Mahat - Divine Mind or Cosmic Intelligence

Manas - outer or sensory aspect of mind

Mantra - seed sounds used for healing or yogic purposes

Marmas - sensitive points on the body

Niyamas - yogic disciplines

Ojas - water on a vital level

Pitta - biological fire humor

Prakriti - nature

Prana - vital force, breath

Pranayama - control or expansion of vital force

Pratyahara - control or introversion of the mind
    and senses

Puja - Hindu rituals

Purusha - inner spirit, Self

Raja Yoga - Integral Yoga system of Patanjali in Yoga
    Sutras

Rajas - quality of action and agitation

Rajasic - of the nature of rajas

Samadhi - absorption

Samana - balancing vital force

Sattva - quality of harmony

Sattvic - of the nature of Sattva

Shakti - power, energy, particular of the deepest level

Shiva - Divine power of peace and transcendence

Tamas - quality of darkness and inertia

Tamasic - of the nature of Tamas

Tanmatras - sensory potentials which are the subtle
    elements (sound, touch, sight, taste, smell)

Tantra - energetic system of working with our higher
    potentials

Tejas - fire on a vital level

Udana - upward moving Prana

Vata - biological air humor

Vayu-another name for Prana or vital force

Vedas - ancient Hindu spiritual system of Self and
    Cosmic knowledge

Vishnu - Divine power of love and protection

Vyana - expansive vital force

Yama - yogic values

Yantras - geometric meditation forms

Yoga - science of reintegration with the universal reality

Herbal Glossary

aloe gel ....Aloe vera
amalaki ....Emblica officinalis
asafetida................Ferula asafetida
ashwagandha ....Withania somnifera
bala ....Sida cordifolia
basil......................Ocinum spp.
bayberry................Myrica spp.
betony ....Stachys betonica
calamus-................Acorus calamus
camomile ....Anthemum nobilis
camphor................Cinnamomum camphor
cardamom ....Elettaria cardamomum
cedar ....Cedrus spp.
champak ....Michelia champaka
chrysanthemum ....Chrysanthemum indicum
cinnamon..............Cinnamomum zeylonica
cloves....................Syzgium aromaticum
damiana ....Turnera aphrodisiaca
elecampane............Inula spp.
ephedra ....Ephedra spp.
eucalyptus ....Eucalyptus sp.
frankincense..........Boswellia carteri
gardenia................Gardenia floribunda
garlic- ....Allium sativa
ginger ....Zingiberis officinalis
gokshura ....Tribulis terrestris
gotu kola ....Hydrocotyle asiatica
guggul..................Commiphora mukul
haritaki ....Terminalia chebula
heena ....Lawsonia alba
honeysuckle..........Lonicera japonica
hops......................Humulus lupulus

hyssop	Hyssop officinalis
iris	Iris sp.
jasmine	Jasminum grandiflorum
jatamansi	Nardostachys jatamansi
kapikacchu	Mucuna pruriens
lady's slipper	Cyripidium pubescens
lavender	Lavendula stoechas
lemon grass	Cymbopogon citratus
licorice	Glycyrrhizzra glabra
lily	Lilum spp.
lotus seeds	Nelumbo nocifera
ma huang	Ephedra sinense
manduka parni	Bacopa monnieri
myrrh	Commiphora myrrha
nutmeg	Myristica fragrans
passion flower	Passiflora incarnata
peppermint	Mentha piperita
pippali	Piper nigrum
plumaria	Plumeria rubra
rose-	Rosa spp.
rosemary	Rosmarinus officinalis
saffron	Crocus sativa
sage	Salvia officinalis
sandalwood	Santalum alba
sesame seeds	Sesamum indica
shankha pushpi	Canscora decussata
shatavari	Asparagus racemosus
shilajit	Asphaltum
skullcap	Scutellaria spp.
spearmint	Mentha spictata
tamarind	Tamarindus indicus
thyme	Thymus vulgaris
valerian	Valeriana spp.

vetivert ....Andropogon muriaticus
vidari ....Ipomoea digitata
wintergreen ....Gaultheria procumbens
yohimbe................Caryanthe yohimbe
zizyphus seeds ......Zizyphus spinosa

BIBLIOGRAPHY

English

Anirvan, *Sri, Antaryoga*, Voice of India, New Delhi, India, 1994.

Anirvan, Sri,. *Buddhiyoga of the Gita and other Essays,* Samata Press, Madras, India, 1990.

Aurobindo, Sri, *Letters on Yoga,* Sri Aurobindo Ashram, Pondicherry, India. Dist. By Lotus Press, Twin Lakes, WI.

Frawley, David, *Astrology of the Seers: A Guide to Hindu/ Vedic Astrology,* Lotus Press, Twin Lakes, WI, 1990.

Frawley, David,. *Ayurvedic Healing, A Comprehensive Guide,* Lotus Press, Twin Lakes, WI. 1989.

Frawley, David, *Beyond The Mind,* Passage Press, Salt Lake City, Utah, 1992.

Frawley, David, *From the River of Heaven: Hindu and Vedic Knowledge for the Modern Age,* Lotus Press, Twin Lakes, WI. 1990.

Frawley, David, *Tantric Yoga and the Wisdom Goddesses: Spiritual Secrets of Ayurveda*, Lotus Press, Twin Lakes, WI. 1994.

Frawley, David and Dr. Vasant Lad, *The Yoga of Herbs,*. Lotus Press, Twin Lakes, WI. 1986.

Lad, Vasant, Dr,. *Ayurveda, The Science of Self-Healing,*. Lotus Press, Twin Lakes, WI. 1984.

Lad, Vasant, Dr. *Ayurvedic Cooking for Self-Healing,*. Ayurvedic Institute, Albuquerque, New Mexico, 1994.

Ranade, Dr. Subhash and Frawley, David *Ayurveda: Nature's Medicine,* Lotus Press, Twin Lakes, WI. 1993.

Yogeshwarananda, Swami, *Science of the Soul,* Yoga Niketan Trust, New Delhi, India, 1992.

Yogeshwarananda, Swami, *Science of the Soul,* Yoga Niketan Trust, New Delhi, India, 1992.

Yogeshwarananda, Swami, *Science of Prana,* Yoga Niketan Trust, New Delhi, India, 1992.

Yukteswar, Sri, *The Holy Science,* Self-Realization Fellowship, Los Angeles, California, 1978.

Sanskrit Texts

Astanga Hridaya of Vagbhatta.

Bhagavad Gita of Sri Krishna.

Caraka Samhita (three volumes). Varanasi, Chowkhamba Sanskrit Series, India.

Daivarata Vaisvamitra, *Chandodarshana.*

Daivarata Vaisvamitra, *Vak Sudha.*

Ganapati Muni, *Uma Sahasram* with commentary by Kapali Sastri.

Mahabharata, Sanskrit, Gita Press, Gorakpur.

Patanjali, *Yoga Sutras* with commentaries of Vacaspati Misra and Vijnana Bhiksu.

Sankhya Karika of Ishvara Krishna with the commentaries of Matharacarya and Samkaracarya.

Satapatha Brahmana

Susruta Samhita

188 Upanishads

Vedantasara

ABOUT THE AUTHOR AND THE AMERICAN INSTITUTE OF VEDIC STUDIES

DAVID FRAWLEY (VAMADEVA SHASTRI)

David Frawley (Vamadeva Shastri) is one of the most respected Vedic teachers (Vedacharyas) in the world today, whose range of study includes Ayurveda, Yoga, Vedanta, Vedic astrology and the ancient Vedas. He is the author of forty published books translated into twenty languages over the last several decades. He has worked with various Vedic and Hindu organizations throughout the world.

Frawley is a rare recipient of the Padma Bhushan Award, the third highest civilian award of the government of India, for his diverse work in the Vedic field. He has a D.Litt. From SVYASA (Swami Vivekananda Yoga Anusandhana Sansthana) the only deemed Yoga university in India, and a second D. Litt. from Avadh University (Ayodhya) in Uttar Pradesh. He was given a National Eminence Award as a Vedacharya from the South Indian Education Society (SIES) in Mumbai. He has been a visiting professor for Sanchi University in Madhya Pradesh and Nalanda University in Bihar.

Frawley is one of the four main advisors of NAMA (National Ayurvedic Medical Association) in the United States, which has honored him as an Ayurvedic doctor. He has been an advisor and Master Educator to the Chopra center since it's founding. He has been a keynote speaker for the ministry of AYUSH India at several conferences. He is an advisor to a number of Ayurvedic schools and organizations worldwide. His books on Ayurveda are among the first published and remain among the most widely used in the field. He has addressed mind and consciousness in several books on Yoga and Vedanta as well.

@drdavidfrawley Facebook
@davidfrawleyved, Twitter

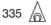

AMERICAN INSTITUTE OF VEDIC STUDIES

DAVID FRAWLEY (VAMADEVA SHASTRI)

Frawley is the director of the American Institute of Vedic Studies (www.vedanet.com), which is an on-line educational center for Vedic Studies for students throughout the world. His wife Yogini Shambhavi Chopra joins him for teaching programs and Yoga retreats, as well offering Vedic astrology consultations. The website hosts more than two hundred original articles by Frawley on Vedic studies and a variety of resources.

The institute offers four on-line courses:

1. Ayurvedic Healing: foundation course in Ayurveda, including the Ayurvedic view of body and mind, constitution, disease and treatment, emphasizing herbal and life-style therapies, since 1988.

2. Yoga, Ayurveda, Mantra and Meditation: foundation course including Ayurveda and Raja Yoga, Yoga Sutras and Sanskrit mantras, Vedanta and consciousness, since 2004.

3. Integral Vedic Counseling: foundation course sharing educational and communication skills and Vedic life guidance relative to all Vedic fields, since 2017.

4. Ayurvedic Astrology: foundation course in Vedic astrology, including the fundamentals of Vedic astrology from birth charts to Muhurta, with special emphasis on the astrology of healing through Ayurveda, since 1985.

For further information contact:
American Institute of Vedic Studies
P.O. Box 8357
Santa Fe, NM 87504-8357

David Frawley (Pandit Vamadeva Shastri), Director
vedicinstitute@gmail.com
www.vedanet.com

INDEX

Abhyanga, 201
Affirmations, 288-289
Agni, 172-173, 233, 316
Ahamkara, 126, 141-142, 318
Air
    Element, 12-13, 62, 190
    Types, 25, 154-155
Ananda, 311
Anandamaya Kosha, 84, 99-100, 309-310
Annamaya Kosha, 84, 99-100, 309-310
Aroma Therapy, 216-221
Aromas, 216-221
Ashtanga Yoga, 263
Association, (Right), 151-152
Astral Plane, 297
Astringent Taste, 192, 198
Astrology, 211
Atman, 98, 126
Awakened Prana, 100-101
Awareness, 8-10, 49, 75
Being, 311
Being-Consciousness-Bliss, 311
Bhakti Yoga, 142
Bitter Taste, 192, 195-196
Bliss, 60, 311
Brahman, 244, 311
Brahmacharya, 266-268
Breath, 25, 100, 270-273
Breathing
    Alternative Nostril, 276
Buddha, 93
Buddhi, 93, 113-116

Buddhism, 4, 253
Causal, 171, 176, 307-312
Chakras, 312-313
Chit, 76, 81, 98, 136
Chitta, 76-79, 81-87, 97-100
Christ, 250- 297
Coconut Oil, 202
Color Therapy, 205-206, 209-210, 213, 287
Compassion, 248, 254
Conscience, 96-97
Consciousness (see Chitta)
    Pure, (see Chit)
Constitutional Types, 15-24, 154-165
Cosmic Consciousness, 80-81, 89, 98, 288
    Life, 182, 231, 259, 289
    Mind, 39, 117, 252
    Person, 311
Counseling, 149
Death, 102, 253, 291, 308
Deep Sleep, 88, 174
Deities, 252-253
Desire, 122
Detoxification, 174-176, 192, 234
Devotion, 244-245, 248, 250
Dharana, 283-284
Dharma, 263-264
Dharmic Living, 259
Dhyana, 289-290
Diet, 150, 170, 186-192, 194-195, 268
    Vegetarian, 39, 191, 268
Divine
    Consciousness, 90, 251
    Father, 81
    Mother, 6

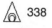
Name, 250-251
Self, 82
Word, 98
Dreams, 88, 174
E.S.P., 121
Earth Element, 64, 190
Ego, 125-133
Elements, 170-171, 190
Emotion, 113-114
Faith, 91
Fire Elements, 13, 190
Fire Types, 13, 18-19, 59-66, 110
Five Senses, 110, 172, 250
Foods, 187, 191, 193-194
Gem Therapy, 205, 211
Gems, 147, 182, 205, 211-216, 333
Ghee, 200-201, 209, 251, 284-285
God, 248-251
God-realization, 134
Goddess, 234, 244, 249, 253
Gods, 32, 117, 250-252
Gunas, 29-35, 41-42, 171
Guru, 98, 104, 154, 128, 250, 289
Hamsa, 273
Hanuman, 253
Heart, 67, 82-83, 90-91
Herbs, 176, 183-186, 195-199
Hessonite, 214
Hinduism, 252-253
Homa, 210
Honey, 200
Ida, 274-276
Incense, 182-201, 216-218
Individual Nature, 86
Insanity, 155, 297

Instinct, 90
Intellect, 94-96
Intelligence, 62, 63, 69, 93-99
Ishvara, 133, 244, 267
Ishvara Pranidhana, 134, 267
Jiva, 132-133, 135-136
Jivatman, 132, 317
Jupitor, 212-214
Kali, 186, 250, 253
Kapha, 11-15, 20-25
Karma, 6-7
Ketu, 213
Krishna, 184, 250, 253
Kundalini, 274, 313
Kwan Yin, 250
Lakshmi, 185, 253
Logos, 98
Love, 90
Mahadeva, 252
Manas, 109-111, 116-117, 119-120, 137-142
Mandalas, 210, 287
Manomaya Kosha, 117, 309
Mantra, 176, 224-226, 230-235, 251
Marmas, 219
Mars, 212-214
Matter, 311
Meditation, 229-230, 285-287, 289-292
Memory, 87-88
Mercury, 212-214
Metals, 215-216
Mind (see Manas)
Mind-Body Medicine, 1, 4, 6
Moon, 184, 212-214
Mustard Oil, 202
Nadis, 231, 273-276

Nasya, 201
Negative Emotions, 89
New Age, 312
Niyamas, 267, 274, 302, 320
Non-possessiveness, 265-266
Non-violence, 265
Oil Massage, 165, 201-203
Ojas, 25-28
OM, 225, 231-233
Organs (Motor), 110-111
Pancha Karma, 203
Paramatman, 135
Perception, 67-68
Pingala, 274-276
Pitta, 11-15, 18-19, 22-25
Planets, 211-213, 244
Prakriti, 128, 171
Prana, 25-28, 100-101, 111-112, 298-299, 314
    Vayus
        Apana, 131, 314, 316
        Prana, 314, 315
        Samana 314, 316
        Udana, 314, 316
        Vyana, 314, 316
Pranamaya Kosha, 309-310
Pratipaksha-Bhavana, 165
Pratyahara, 176, 272, 280-283
Prayer, 251
Psychoanalysis, 5, 300
Puja, 250
Pungent Taste, 196
Rahu, 213
Rajas, 30-36, 38-41
Rama, 184, 253
Reason, 63, 67

Rejuventatives, 199
Relationships, 245-246
Rituals, 250-251
Rudra, 186, 253
Salty Taste, 197
Samadhi, 88-89
Samskaras, 86
Samyama, 264
Sarasvati, 234
Satsanga, 153
Sattva, 30-36, 38-42
Sattvic Diet, 190-192, 194
    Prana, 100, 299
    Samskara, 301
Saturn, 212-214
Sedatives, 199
Self
    Discipline, 122
    Esteem, 214
    Higher, 66, 136-137
    Inquiry, 142, 257
    Realization, 5
    Sense, 131
    Study, 268
Sense Mind, 66-69, 109, 112, 119
Sesame Oil, 201-202
Sex, 265-266
Shakti, 244, 274
Shiva, 6, 185, 233
Soul, 65-66, 132-137
Sound, 227-228, 288
Sour, 198
Speech, 105, 223-224
Surrender, 247
Sushumna, 273-274

Sweating, 175-176, 198
Tai Chi, 184
Tamas, 30-36, 38-41
Tantra, 4-6
Tara, 184, 250
Taste, 192-193, 195-198
Tejas, 25-28, 85, 100
Therapy
    Balancing, 71, 150, 165
    Spiritual, 243-263, 291-305
    Sublte, 205-221
Therapists, 149-168
Three Doshas, 175, 183, 203
Three Humors, 22, 194, 215, 217
Three Vital Essences, 25-27, 85, 217
Tibetan Buddhism, 253
Tinctures, 198, 200, 212, 219
Tonics, 196, 198-199
Vata, 11-16, 22-25 (see Prana)
Vata-Kapha, 22, 164
Vata-Pitta, 22, 162-163
Vedanta, 4, 135-136
Vedic Astrology, 211
Venus, 212, 214
Vijnanamaya Kosha, 99, 309
Vishnu, 185, 321, 329, 333
Vision, 121-122
Vrittis, 309-310
Water Element, 13-14, 63-64
Water Types, 20-22
Will, 85, 101-103, 122, 247
Yamas, 264-265, 274, 302
Yantras, 238, 252, 284, 287

Yoga, 259-305
    Eight Limbs of, 263, 302
    Hatha, 184
    Jnana, 142
    Raja, 320
    Sutras, 259, 263, 291

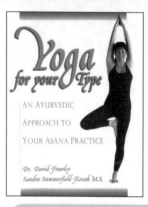
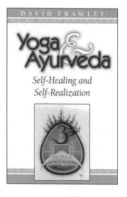

David Frawley Titles

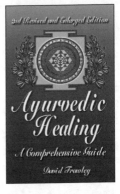

Ayurvedic Healing
A Comprehensive Guide,
2nd Revised and Enlarged Edition
David Frawley
468 pp pb • $22.95 • ISBN: 978-0-9149-5597-9

Ayurvedic Healing presents Ayurvedic treatments for over eighty common diseases and ailments, from the common cold to cancer. This extraordinary manual of ayurvedic health care offers the ancient system of mind-body medicine to the modern reader. Treatment methods include traditional approaches using diet, herbs, oils, gems, mantra and meditation for today's health concerns. Learn empowering Ayurvedic lifestyle practices and daily health considerations for your personal mind-body type! Revised and expanded edition.

"Ayurvedic Healing provides a practical how-to-do-it approach rather than another theoretical treatise. Both the general public as well as professional practitioners will welcome this book."
— **Michael Tierra**, Author of *The Way of Herbs, The Natural Remedy Bible*

"David Frawley is among the leading Ayurvedic experts in the Western world. He has immeasurably contributed to our awareness of the value of Ayurveda. Ayurvedic Healing will be a classic."
— **Deepak Chopra, M.D.**, Author of *The Seven Spiritual Laws of Success*

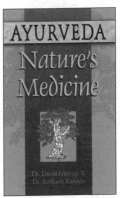

Ayurveda, Nature's Medicine
David Frawley & Dr. Subhash Ranade
368 pp pb • $19.95 • ISBN: 978-0-9149-5595-5

Ayurveda, Nature's Medicine details India's extraordinary natural healing traditions rooted in five thousand years of practice. The Ayurvedic "science of life" is a mind-body system that includes physical, psychological and spiritual healing. This book explains Ayurvedic approaches to all levels of wellness, including diagnostic and treatment methods, and the healing techniques of diet, herbs, yoga and meditation. It shares the wisdom of daily and seasonal regimes for optional health and vitality, along with lifestyle recommendations concerning exercise, sexuality and diet.

Ayurveda, Nature's Medicine covers the material found in India's institutions of higher learning for foreign students in two-year programs. This wealth of information reveals the secret healing powers of nature and the vitality of our life-force, or prana. This is essential reading for those interested in Ayurveda and the foundation of mind-body medicine.

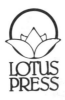

David Frawley Titles

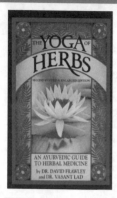

The Yoga of Herbs
Ayurvedic Guide to Herbal Medicine
2nd Revised and Enlarged Edition
David Frawley & Dr. Vasant Lad
288 pp • $15.95 • ISBN: 978-0-9415-2424-7

For the first time, here is a detailed explanation and classification of herbs, using the ancient system of Ayurveda. More than 270 herbs are listed, with 108 herbs explained in detail. Included are many of the most commonly used western herbs with a profound Ayurvedic perspective. Important Chinese and special Ayurvedic herbs are introduced. Beautiful diagrams and charts, as well as detailed glossaries, appendices and index are included.

"This book is a fresh application of Ayurvedic principles to Western herbs. As such it stands as a landmark in the development of Western herbology, allowing a deeper blending of Eastern and Western herbology."
— **Paul Bergner**, East West Journal

"The Yoga of Herbs provides a fascinating and readable look at Ayurveda. This book acts as a key, unlocking the mysteries of Eastern philosophies and medical practices. One views the energies and actions of American herbs with a fresh perspective after reading this valuable, timeless volume. Highly recommended."
— **Stephen Foster**, Herbalist, Author

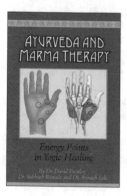

Ayurveda and Marma Therapy
David Frawley, Dr. Subhash Ranade & Dr. Lele Avinash
272 pp • $21.95 • ISBN: 978-0-9409-8559-9

Marmas are special Ayurvedic energy points on the body, connected to the chakras and nadis of Yoga. These energy points can be worked to direct our Prana, or vital energy, towards healing and balance between mind and body. Marma therapy is one of the great tools of Yogic and Ayurvedic healing, and a knowledge of this system is important for practitioners of either modality.

Ayurveda and Marma Therapy clearly describes the 107 main marma points in location, properties and usage. It details treatment methods such as massage, aromas, herbs and yoga practices. Recognized as the first book in marma therapy published in the West, it is an essential reference guide for all students of Yoga, Ayurveda, massage or natural healing.

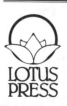

These books are available at bookstores and natural food stores nationwide.
To order a copy directly visit **LotusPress.com**

For more information or other ways to order
e-mail: **lotuspress@lotuspress.com** or call 262-889-8561

Lotus Press is the publisher of a wide range of books in the field of alternative health, including Ayurveda, Chinese medicine, herbology, aromatherapy, Reiki and energetic healing modalities.

David Frawley Titles

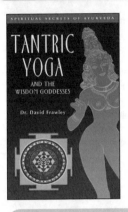

Tantric Yoga
and the Wisdom Goddesses
David Frawley
260 pp • $16.95 • ISBN: 978-0-9102-6139-5

"Tantric Yoga and the Wisdom Goddesses is an excellent introduction to the essence of Hindu Tantrism. The author discusses all the major concepts and offers valuable corrections for many existing misconceptions. He also introduces the reader to the core Tantric practices of meditation and mantra recitation, focusing on the ten Wisdom Goddesses."
- Synopsis by **Georg Feuerstein**, yogic scholar and Indologist.

"Dr. David Frawley is one of the most important scholars of Ayurveda and Vedic Science today. I have gained great personal insight from his work and have great respect and admiration for his knowledge, and for the lucid way in which he has expounded the ancient wisdom of the Vedas. Anyone who is exposed to Dr. Frawley's work is bound to not only become more knowledgeable but wiser."
— **Deepak Chopra, M.D.**

"David Frawley in his book Tantric Yoga and the Wisdom Goddesses successfully removes the misunderstandings regarding Tantra which have clouded the vision of under informed students of Tantra. His presentation is the first time that English readers have an opportunity to learn about the Ten Mahavidyas, the central doctrine and practice of Shakta Tantricism in great detail. The uniqueness of the book lies in how the author pulls together Tantric and Ayurvedic sciences in a manner which one can practice in one's daily life."
— **Pandit Rajmani Tigunait**, Himalayan Institute

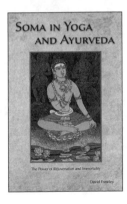

Soma in Yoga and Ayurveda:
The Power of Rejuvenation and Immortality
David Frawley
392 pp • $19.95 • ISBN: 978-0-9406-7621-3

Going back to the vision of the Vedic Seers, David Frawley reveals the secret of Soma for body, mind and spirit, with its implications from diet and herbs to pranayama, mantra and meditation. His new analysis of Soma is practical, comprehensive and deeply insightful so that you can bring the secret power of Soma to all aspects of your life and to the world as a whole.

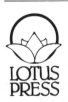

David Frawley Titles

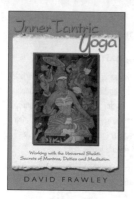

Inner Tantric Yoga
Frawley, David
280 pp • $19.95 • ISBN: 978-0-9406-7650-3

Inner Tantric Yoga presents the deeper tradition of Tantra, its multidimensional vision of the Divine and its transformative practices of mantra and meditation that take us far beyond the outer models of how Tantra is usually presented today. The book can expand your horizons about masculine and feminine energies, Self and world, universe and the Absolute into a living experience of the Infinite and Eternal both within and around you.

"With *Inner Tantric Yoga*, David Frawley reminds us that we have, hidden within our own deeper awareness, wonderful Gods and Goddesses in embryo who have but one intention: to bring the sacred back into our lives."
— **Deepak Chopra and David Simon**, the Chopra Center for Wellbeing

"Vamadeva (Dr. Frawley) is a living rishi who guides his students to the fullest scope of yogic insight and realization. His boook weaves Tantra, Veda and Yoga, Shakti and Shiva, into a magnificent tapestry of wisdom, beauty and delight."
— **Shambhavi Chopra**, author of *Yogini, Unfolding the Goddess Within*

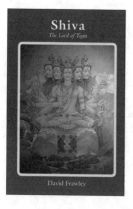

Shiva
The Lord of Yoga
David Frawley
296 pp • $19.95 • ISBN: 978-0-9406-7629-9

Lord Shiva is the personification of all the main practices of Yoga, as the origin and ruling power over asana, prana, mantra, inner seeing and meditation. He is the ultimate Yoga guru reflecting the highest Self-awareness. Yet this centrality of Shiva in Yoga is rarely understood and utilized. The current book unfolds the presence, light, energy and consciousness of the Supreme Shiva to take us all beyond all death and duality.

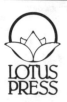

These books are available at bookstores and natural food stores nationwide.
To order a copy directly visit **LotusPress.com**

For more information or other ways to order
e-mail: **lotuspress@lotuspress.com** or call 262-889-8561

Lotus Press is the publisher of a wide range of books in the field of alternative health, including Ayurveda, Chinese medicine, herbology, aromatherapy, Reiki and energetic healing modalities.